Time-Saving Fitness: Revitalize Your 40+ Body with 5-Minute Workouts

BILLIE .R. FLORES

1

Table of contents:

Introduction: Recovering Your Imperativeness
Embracing Wellness in Your 40s and Then some
the Force of 5-Minute Exercises.

Introduction:

Recovering Your Imperativeness

Embracing Wellness in Your 40s and Then some the Force of 5-Minute Exercises.

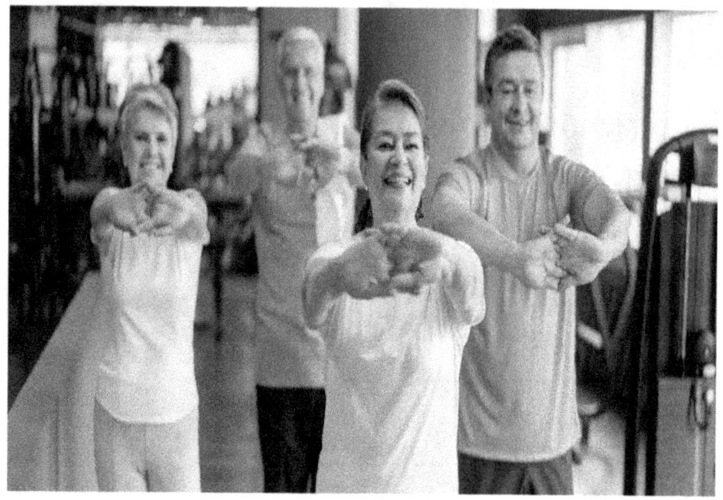

- Recuperating Your Essentialness: Embrace Life's Subsequent Demonstration

In the terrific story of life, the 40s and past are in many cases portrayed as the dusk years, when essentialness fades, and the sundown years start. Notwithstanding, imagine a scenario in which I let you know that these years could be the beginning of a lively new section loaded up with energy, excitement, and vitality. Now is the right time to break the generalization that maturing implies dialing back and embrace the idea of "Recuperating Your Noteworthiness."

- The Legend of the Emotional meltdown

A significant number of us have caught wind of the scandalous emotional meltdown, a time of assumed strife and discontent that strikes when we arrive in our 40s or 50s. It's not unexpectedly portrayed as when individuals go with rash choices, purchase sports vehicles, or leave on nonsensical undertakings. Yet, imagine a scenario in which we saw this stage as a novel open door rather than an emergency.

- Embracing Change

Recuperating your essentialness starts with embracing change. In all actuality, life is dynamic, and change is the main consistent. Instead of opposing it, we should greet it wholeheartedly. Our bodies and brains might be unique in relation to what they were in our 20s, yet that doesn't mean they're any less competent.

They can be much more exceptional, as a matter of fact.

- The Force of 5-Minute Wellness

Perhaps the main confusion about maturing is that you really want long stretches of exhausting exercises to remain in shape. In any case, imagine a scenario where I let you know that you can launch your excursion to criticality in only 5 minutes every day. Indeed, you read that accurately — 5 minutes! There's no need to focus on amount; it's about consistency and quality.

- Filling Your Essentialness

Nourishment assumes a vital part in your journey to recuperate your importance. There's actually no need to focus on eating less junk food or hardship; it's tied in with sustaining your body and brain. For getting healthy, the kind of food you eat is everything, so why not pick food sources that strengthen you, give supported energy, and advance generally prosperity?

- Careful Development and Stress Decrease

Your essentialness isn't just about actual imperativeness; it's about mental and close to home force as well. Integrating care rehearses into your day to day schedule can assist you with overseeing pressure, increment strength, and develop an uplifting perspective on life. It's tied in with remaining focused and associated with your internal identity.

- Following Advancement and Remaining Roused

Recuperating your hugeness is an excursion, not an objective. Laying out reasonable objectives, keeping tabs on your development, and praising your accomplishments are crucial parts of remaining roused. The delight lies in the excursion, in addition to the final product.

- Beating Normal Difficulties

No excursion is without its difficulties. From a throbbing painfulness to carving out opportunity in your bustling timetable, obstructions will show up. Yet, these are not detours; they are venturing stones. Each challenge you conquer carries you one bit nearer to recuperating your significance.

- Rousing Stories of Criticalness

To really trust in the force of recuperating your vitality, look no farther than the people who have strolled this way before you. Their moving stories act as a demonstration of the way that age is only a number. You'll track down stories of change, versatility, and the sheer assurance to make every moment count.

- Decision: A Better, More joyful You

Recuperating your hugeness isn't tied in with recovering lost youth; it's tied in with embracing the present and future with great affection. It's tied in with expressing yes to life, esteeming each second, and understanding that the best is on the way. Your criticalness isn't something you've lost; it's a holding up thing to be revealed, supported, and celebrated.

All in all, "Recuperating Your Significance" isn't a legend or a transient thought. It's an unmistakable, feasible reality. It's tied in with understanding that life doesn't end at 40; it's simply beginning.

In this way, require that 5-minute step towards a better, more joyful you. Embrace change, fuel your significance, practice care, remain propelled, conquer difficulties, and be roused by the individuals who have made ready. Life's subsequent demonstration is your chance to hit one out of the ballpark, and the world is your stage. Hold onto it, love it, and recuperate your importance with each breath you

Chapter 1:

The 5- Minute Wellness:

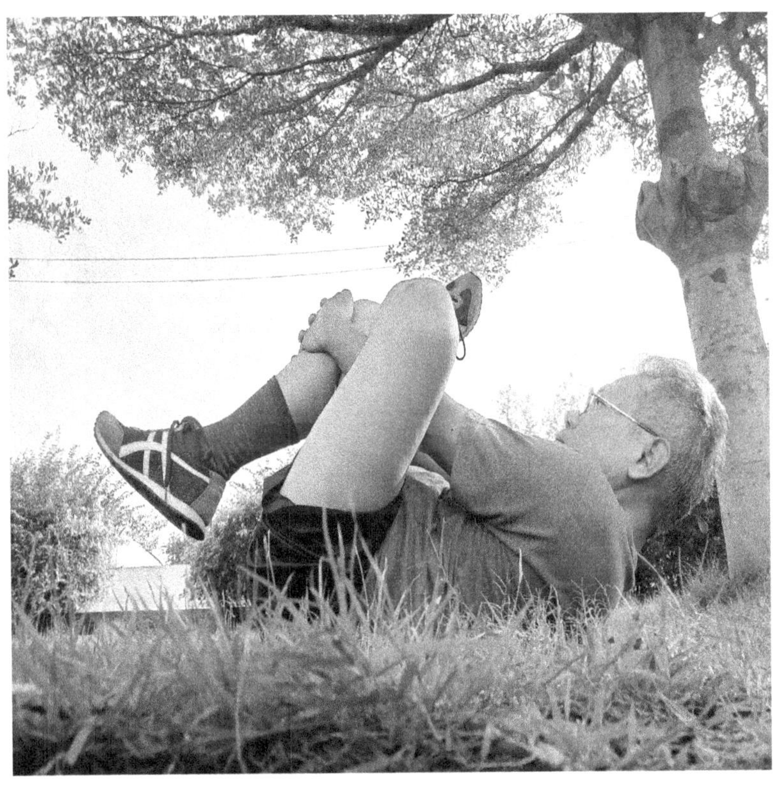

Unrest 5- nanosecond Good Agitation Touch off Your Good Upset Picture this An actuality where you do not have to commit hours to the exercise center, spend a fortune on popular weight control plans, or pursue mode good patterns to be sound and feel unconceivable.

All effects considered, fantasize an introductory, progressive idea that changes your substance in only 5 twinkles per day. Drink to the" 5- nanosecond Good fermentation," a development that's changing lives and testing all that you assumed you had some mindfulness of good and imperativeness.

Breaking the Chains of Show For a really long time, we have been molded to accept that genuine health requires vast long ages of sweat, penance, and battle. The" 5- nanosecond Good Agitation" is then to free you from that enervating worldview.

It's tied in with understanding that significant changes can appear from little, predictable conditioning. Only 5 twinkles every day, and you will be on the way to a better, more lively you. The Force of Model Propensities Consider it What might you at any point achieve in only 5 twinkles? Mix some espresso? Look at virtual entertainment?

Or on the other hand might you at some point use those precious twinkles to change your life?" The 5- nanosecond Good fermentation" presents the idea of atomic propensities — little, sensible changes you can integrate fluently into your everyday diurnal practice.

These small, steady advances amass over the long haul, egging shocking issues. Speedy and important Exercises factual heartiness constantly feels like an insolvable test, particularly for those with engaged lives.

Yet, imagine a script in which you could negotiate noteworthy heartiness acquired in only 5 twinkles. Short, serious exercises planned by specialists can help your digestion, develop fiber, and work on cardiovascular good.

Express farewell to expansive exercise center meetings and hi to the" 5- Minute Wellness Upheaval." Aliment Simplified Aliment need not be a maze of confounding eating rules and complex regale plans.

With the" 5- Minute Health Agitation," you will figure out how to make expertise, acclimated opinions snappily.

Find simple fashions, fast regale fix procedures, and the force of careful eating — each in only 5 twinkles. Care for Mental Lucidity In a world loaded up with interruptions and stress, your cerebral substance is more critical than any other time.

The" 5- Minute Health Turmoil" presents care procedures that give limpidness, attention, and stress relief. These terse day to day practices will help you with exploring life's difficulties with beauty and strength.

Following Advancement and Remaining Roused A vital element of the" 5- Minute Health Turmoil" is remaining focused. Figure out how to put forth doable objects, screen your advancement, and remain propelled on your excursion.

Celebrate little triumphs and substantiate the change by extending each 5- nanosecond scrap in turn. Supporting excrescence Embrace your mars and recommend your extraordinary excursion to good. The" 5- Minute Health Turmoil" perceives that life is chaotic, and that's entirely alright.

It's about progress, not flawlessness. With only 5 twinkles, you can ameliorate effects significantly in your good and bliss. Join the Unrest Could it be said that you're set to join the" 5- nanosecond Good Agitation"? It's a development that's comprehensive, engaging, and open to all.

No matter what your age, heartiness, position, or schedule, you can touch off your good uneasiness in only 5 twinkles every day. End Your 5- nanosecond Excursion to Health The" 5- nanosecond Good fermentation" is in excess of an idea; it's a source of alleviation.

It shakes effects up, disturbs the standard way of thinking, and enables you to assume command over your substance.

runner farewell to the old guidelines and embrace the 5- nanosecond change in perspective that will change your life. Prepare to light your good worries — each 5- nanosecond move toward turn. Your good is breaking, and it's nearer than you suspect.

2. Separating the Obstructions to Exercise:

Isolating the Impediments to Exercise: Release Your Internal Wellness Champion

Chasing better wellbeing and essentialness, barely any things are basically as all inclusive as the craving to routinely work-out. However, regardless of our best aims, endless deterrents frequently disrupt the general flow of accomplishing our wellness objectives. Now is the right time to deal with these boundaries directly, to overcome them, and release your inward wellness hero. We should investigate how you can begin isolating the hindrances to exercise and clear the way to a better, more joyful you.

- The Covert Saboteurs

Envision wellness as an impressive palace, and your objective as the fortune inside. Presently, picture the impediments as covert saboteurs, attempting to hold you back from arriving at your fortune. These impediments can take many structures:

Time Imperatives: The persevering walk of our regular routines frequently pretty much rules out work out. Work, family, and different responsibilities can make it difficult to cut out time for exercises.

Absence of Inspiration: In some cases, it's basically hard to marshal the inspiration expected to consistently work-out. The lounge chair looks more welcoming than the exercise center, and dawdling dominates.

Injury and Torment: Actual constraints, like wounds and ongoing agony, can be significant checks. Anxiety toward compounding these circumstances can keep us from getting dynamic.

Climate Burdens: In the event that you're an open air fan, terrible weather conditions can be a critical hindrance. Downpour, snow, or outrageous intensity can make practice less engaging.

Rec center Terrorizing: The scary environment of certain exercise centers can be a huge boundary. The anxiety toward judgment or feeling awkward keeps numerous from the weight room.

- The Craft of Deterrent Partition

Fortunately these impediments are not impervious obstructions. They are obstacles that you can defeat with the right methodologies. This is the way to begin isolating them:

Focus on and Timetable: The way to handle time imperatives is to focus on exercise and timetable it like some other significant arrangement. Close off committed exercise time in your schedule, and treat it as non-debatable.

Put forth Moving Objectives: Inspiration frequently winds down when you don't have clear, rousing objectives. Set explicit, feasible wellness objectives that energize you. Whether it's running a 5k or dominating a difficult yoga present, having an objective will light your inspiration.

Pay attention to Your Body: On the off chance that wounds or agony are keeping you down, it's vital to pay attention to your body. Counsel a medical care proficient or an actual specialist to foster an activity plan that works for yourself and addresses your particular requirements.

Weatherproof Your Exercise: Weather conditions won't be a reason any longer. Put resources into adaptable exercise gear or investigate indoor activity choices like home exercises, yoga, or indoor pools.

Find an Agreeable Wellness Space: In the event that the rec center climate is scaring, look for options. Think about more modest, less jam-packed rec centers, open air parks, or virtual wellness classes where you can practice serenely.

- Local area and Backing

Isolating impediments becomes simpler when you're in good company on your excursion. Search out help and local area:

Responsibility Accomplices: Cooperate with a companion or relative who shares your wellness objectives. Having somebody to practice with and consider you responsible can be a unique advantage.

Online People group: Join online wellness gatherings or discussions where you can associate with similar people, share encounters, and track down inspiration and exhortation.

Proficient Direction: Consider working with a fitness coach or wellness mentor who can fit an exercise plan to your requirements and give master direction.

End: Release Your Inward Wellness Hero

As you leave on your excursion to isolate the hindrances to work out, recollect that each step in the right direction is a triumph.

You're not combating alone; you're joining a worldwide local area of people focused on better lives.

With the right mentality, techniques, and backing, you can release your inward wellness fighter and overcome these deterrents, each exercise in turn.

Your wellbeing and essentialness anticipate on the opposite side of these hindrances, and the fortune is yours for the taking.

3. Why 5 twinkles Can fully change you:

Why 5 Twinkles Can Completely Change You Embrace the Force of Atomic Changes In the speedy hurricane of our regular routines, misgauging the effect of only five twinkles is simple. Still, inside these temporary twinkles lies a striking power — a power that can completely ameliorate you.

Now is the ideal time to embrace the idea of atomic changes and open the capability of those precious five twinkles.

The Enchantment of Atomic Changes You may consider," Might five twinkles at any point truly have an effect?" The response is a resonating yes! Atomic changes, the little and predictable changes we make in only five- nanosecond accruals, act structure blocks that can reshape your life.

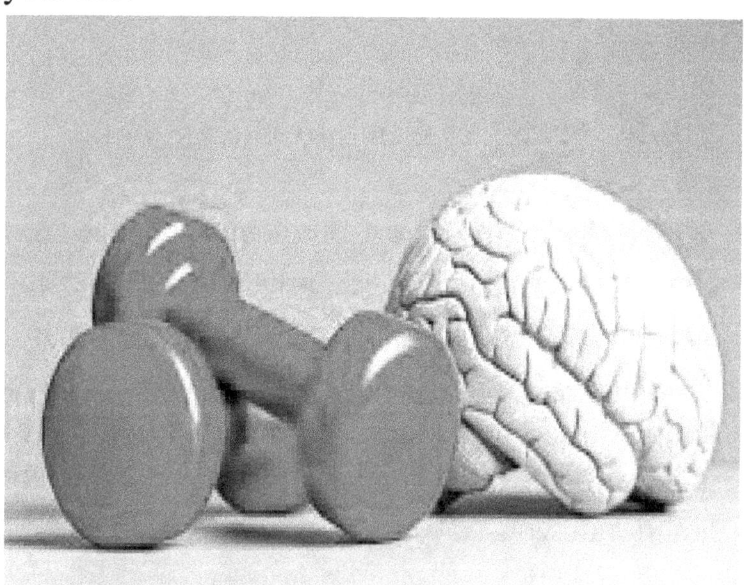

That is the reason they're so important. Reachability Five twinkles is highly doable, indeed in the most active of calendars. It's a gauged down lump of time that anybody can cut out from their day, anyhow of how furious. thickness The way to progress in any undertaking is thickness.

Atomic changes permit you to be steady in your trials, as they're sensible and not overpowering. Force Little palms gather speed. At the point when you witness positive change in only five twinkles, you are bound to do and try and extend your trials. Low Pressure Five twinkles convey negligible strain.

There is a compelling reason to contribute hours or anticipate fantastic issues incontinently. This makes the cycle not so important scary but rather more agreeable. Areas of Change The nobility of five- nanosecond model changes is that they can be applied to different corridor of your life Wellness A speedy eruption of exertion or extending for five twinkles can steadily work on your factual heartiness, support energy situations, and ameliorate by and large good. Care: Go through five twinkles daily in contemplation, profound breathing, or reflection.

This training can lessen pressure, further develop attention, and encourage profound substance.

Learning Devote five twinkles to gaining some new useful knowledge constantly. After some time, you will gather important information and capacities. Association Bear only five twinkles to clean up a little space or make a plan for the day. This little exertion can prompt a more coordinated and effective life. Connections Put five twinkles in associating with musketeers and family.

shoot a sincere communication or take part in a short, significant discussion to support connections.

Embracing Model Changes To rig the force of five twinkles and substantiate the extraordinary change it can bring, suppose about the coexisting advances Set Clear points Fete the aspect of your life you need to get to the coming position.

Be unequivocal about what you need to negotiate in only five twinkles every day. Make an Everyday practice Integrate your five-nanosecond model change into your day to day daily schedule. It may veritably well be during your morning schedule,mid-day break, or before sleep time.

Track Progress Keep a journal or use the following operation to record your everyday trials and results.

Seeing your enhancement will goad you. Observe Little triumphs Fete and recommend your accomplishments, anyhow of how minor they might appear. Each step relies on your excursion of change.

Remain protean Be adaptable and open to changing your atomic changes depending on the situation. On the off chance that one strategy is not working, probe different choices until you find what suits you stylish.

End Embrace the Force of Five twinkles The ensuing time you end up with an redundant five twinkles, do not excuse it as insignificant. All effects considered, flash back it as a chance for change.

Whether you need to work on your factual heartiness, internal substance, connections, or some other part of your life, recollect that five twinkles can completely transfigure you.

Embrace the influence of atomic changes, and watch as those little, predictable trials gather into a life that's further extravagant, better, and more satisfying than you at any point envisaged.

Chapter 2:

1. A Reasonable Way to deal with Wellbeing:

A Sensible Method for managing Prosperity: Equilibrium, Progress, and Taking care of oneself

In a world that frequently lauds outrageous weight control plans, extreme gym routines, and convenient solutions, it's reviving to find a sensible method for managing prosperity. This approach champions balance, continuous advancement, and the fundamental act of taking care of oneself. Now is the ideal time to investigate how you can set out on an excursion to better well being and satisfaction without losing your mental soundness simultaneously.

- Difficult exercise: The Way to Practical Prosperity

Balance is the foundation of a sensible way to deal with prosperity.

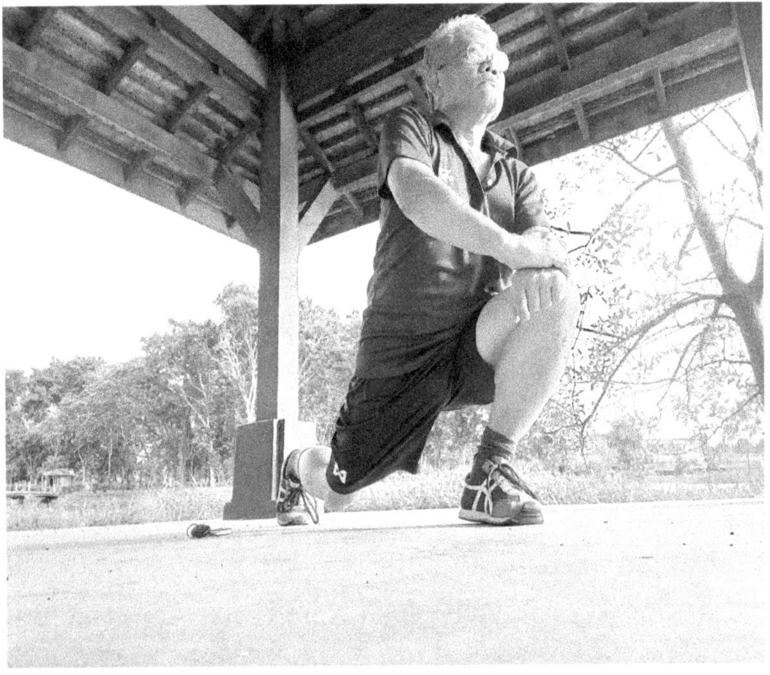

It's tied in with perceiving that you don't have to swing starting with one outrageous then onto the next to be solid. All things being equal, hold back nothing mix of the accompanying components:

Nourishment: As opposed to buying into inflexible weight control plans, center around adjusted eating. Partake in a wide assortment of food varieties, including natural products, vegetables, lean proteins, and entire grains. Indulge yourself once in a while without culpability — everything no doubt revolves around balance.

Work out: Exercise is crucial, however it doesn't need to be tiresome. Integrate exercises you really appreciate into your everyday practice, whether it's moving, climbing, or yoga. Hold back nothing but driving yourself to the limits.

Mental Prosperity: Focus on your emotional wellness similarly as much as your actual wellbeing. Practice care, participate in unwinding methods, and look for help when required. It's OK to request help.

Rest and Recuperation: Satisfactory rest is fundamental for generally speaking prosperity. Guarantee you get sufficient quality rest, and permit yourself personal time to re-energize.

Workaholic behavior can cause more damage than great.

- Progress, Not Flawlessness

One of the most sensible parts of prosperity is embracing progress, not flawlessness. In a world that frequently requests moment results, it's memorable that enduring change requires some investment. This is the way you can gain ground a piece of your excursion:

Put forth Practical Objectives: Characterize feasible, reasonable objectives for yourself. Separate them into more modest, reasonable advances. Commend every achievement en route.

Consistency Is Critical: It's smarter to practice modestly a few times each week than to stretch yourself to the edge for a brief time frame. Consistency bests power.

Gain from Difficulties: Be encouraged by misfortunes or infrequent extravagances. They are a piece of life. What's fundamental is the means by which you quickly return and push ahead.

Measure Past the Scale: Your advancement reaches out past the number on a scale. Consider how you feel, your energy levels, and your general feeling of prosperity. These variables matter similarly to such an extent, while possibly not more.

- The Craft of Taking care of oneself

Taking care of oneself isn't an extravagance; it's a need for a sensible way to deal with prosperity. Dealing with yourself isn't self centered; it's an establishment whereupon you can construct a better and more joyful life. Here are some taking care of oneself practices to consolidate:

Focus on "Personal" Time: Commit minutes in your day exclusively for yourself. Whether it's perusing a book, scrubbing down, or basically partaking in some tea, these minutes are fundamental for revival.

Put down Stopping points: Figure out how to say no as the need should arise. Limits safeguard your significant investment, guaranteeing you have enough for yourself.

Social Associations: Support your connections. Investing energy with friends and family, sharing encounters, and offering backing to each other can fundamentally affect your feeling of prosperity.

Look for Proficient Assistance: In the event that you're battling with physical or psychological wellness issues, go ahead and provide proficient assistance. It's a sensible and capable method for really focusing on yourself.

- Determination: A Sensible Way to Prosperity

In a world frequently loaded up with outrageous arrangements and impractical commitments, a sensible way to deal with prosperity stands apart as both reasonable and compelling. Embrace balance in all parts of your life, center around progress as opposed flawlessly, and focus on taking care of oneself as a non-debatable piece of your daily practice. This way to deal with prosperity isn't about easy routes; it's tied in with making an economical, satisfying, and sound life that you can appreciate long into the future.

2. Sustenance: Energizing Your 40+ Excursion:

Food: Stimulating Your 40+ Journey

Life at 40 and past is a surprising excursion — a period of self-disclosure, freshly discovered insight, and the opportunity to carry on with life based on your conditions. However, it's likewise a stage when your body and brain request some additional consideration. Enter the craft of food — an idea that can really empower your 40+ journey, changing it into a dynamic experience loaded up with imperativeness and prosperity.

- Feeding the Body

Food starts with feeding your body from the back to front. It's tied in with understanding that what you put into your body assumes a critical part by the way you feel and capability. This is the way to excel at food in your 40s and then some:

Adjusted Sustenance: Your eating routine ought to be an amicable mix of supplements, including organic products, vegetables, lean proteins, entire grains, and solid fats. Center around entire, natural food sources, and limit sweet, handled things.

Hydration: Remaining satisfactorily hydrated turns out to be much more basic as you age. Hold back nothing to 8 glasses of water a day and cutoff sweet beverages.

Segment Control: Focus on segment sizes. Your digestion might dial back, so be aware of calorie admission to keep a sound weight.

Careful Eating: Food isn't just about what you eat; it's about how you eat. Practice careful eating by appreciating each chomp and focusing on your body's craving and totality signals.

Supplementation: Talk with a medical services proficient to decide whether enhancements like nutrients and minerals are important to fill any dietary holes.

- Development and Adaptability

Supporting your imperativeness in your 40s and past likewise includes keeping your body dynamic and adaptable. This is the way to accomplish that:

Customary Activity: Hold back nothing 150 minutes of moderate-force oxygen consuming movement each week, like energetic strolling, swimming, or moving. Integrate strength preparing activities to keep up with bulk.

Adaptability and Equilibrium: Yoga and extending schedules assist with further developing adaptability and equilibrium, diminishing the gamble of injury.

Rest and Recuperation: Give your body a satisfactory chance to rest and recuperate between exercises. Focus on rest to help by and large wellbeing and prosperity.

- Care and Stress Decrease

Food isn't just about actual wellbeing; it's additionally about sustaining your psychological and profound prosperity:

Care Practices: Take part in care contemplation, profound breathing activities, or care based pressure decrease projects to oversee pressure and advance mental clearness.

Stress Decrease: Distinguish stressors in your day to day existence and find proactive ways to diminish them. This might include defining limits, looking for help, or making way of life changes.

Social Association: Develop significant connections and participate in friendly exercises that give pleasure and satisfaction to your life.

- Wellbeing Check-Ups
- Standard health check-ups are a fundamental part of food in your 40s and then some:

Clinical Screenings: Keep awake to-date with suggested clinical screenings and tests for conditions, for example, hypertension, cholesterol, diabetes, and malignant growth.

Medical services Group: Construct a medical care group that incorporates an essential consideration doctor and experts to address explicit wellbeing needs.

Stand by listening to Your Body: Focus on your body's signs. On the off chance that something doesn't feel right or on the other hand assuming you experience uncommon side effects, look for clinical counsel quickly.

- A Comprehensive Methodology

Food isn't just about individual parts; it's a comprehensive way to deal with your general prosperity. It's tied in with perceiving that your physical, mental, and close to home wellbeing are interconnected, and they all assume a part in your excursion through your 40s and then some.

- End: Invigorating Your 40+ Trip

Food is the fuel that can control your 40+ trip higher than ever. By supporting your body with adjusted sustenance, remaining dynamic and adaptable, rehearsing care, and focusing on ordinary well being check-ups, you can embrace this period of existence with imperativeness and energy.

Your 40s and past can be the most lively, satisfying long periods of your excursion, and everything starts with the craft of food.

Thus, support your body, brain, and soul, and let the experience of your 40+ years be one loaded up with vast energy and prosperity.

3. The Significance of Rest and Recuperation:

The Meaning of Rest and Recovery: Re-energizing Your Life

In our quick moving, determined worker world, rest and recovery frequently take a secondary lounge to efficiency and accomplishment. In any case, the meaning of rest and recovery couldn't possibly be more significant. It's not simply about enjoying some time off; it's tied in with restoring your body, psyche, and soul, and it assumes an urgent part in your general prosperity and achievement.

- The Rest-Recovery Association
- Rest and recovery are naturally associated however fill various needs:

Rest: Rest alludes to the demonstration of enjoying some time off or stopping from physical or mental action. A transitory relief permits your body and mind to recuperate from weakness, both physical and mental.

Recovery: Recovery, then again, is a more extensive idea enveloping the reclamation and recuperation of your general wellbeing and prosperity. A more extensive cycle includes rest as well as different practices and way of life decisions that help your body's regular mending systems.

- Actual Restoration

Rest and recovery are fundamental for your actual wellbeing and essentialness. Here's the reason:

Muscle Fix: During rest, your body fixes and constructs muscle tissue, which is pivotal for keeping up with strength and usefulness, particularly as you age.

Insusceptible Framework Backing: A very much refreshed body has a more grounded resistant framework, better prepared to ward off contaminations and sicknesses.

Chemical Equilibrium: Satisfactory rest controls chemicals, including those liable for hunger and digestion, advancing a better body piece.

Injury Recuperation: Rest is fundamental for mending wounds, whether they are sports-related or regular strains and injuries.

- Mental Restoration

- Your brain helps similarly as much from rest and recovery:

Stress Decrease: Enjoying reprieves and rehearsing unwinding strategies during rest periods can bring down feelings of anxiety, further developing your generally speaking mental prosperity.

Upgraded Concentration and Innovativeness: Rest permits your cerebrum to re-energize, prompting further developed focus, critical thinking, and inventiveness.

Profound Strength: Sufficient rest directs state of mind and close to home dependability, making you stronger notwithstanding life's difficulties.

Memory Combination: While you rest, your cerebrum processes and solidifies recollections, upgrading your capacity to hold data.

- Difficult exercise

Accomplishing a harmony among action and rest can be testing, however it's critical for supporting your wellbeing and efficiency:

Day to day Rest: Integrate brief breaks into your everyday daily practice. A couple of moments of profound breathing or extending can invigorate your brain and body.

Quality Rest: Focus on rest by laying out a customary rest plan and establishing an agreeable rest climate. Go for long stretches of serene rest every evening.

Booked Recovery: Plan times of more expanded rest and recovery, for example, ends of the week away or get-aways. Detach from work and innovation during these times.

Careful Practices: Take part in care reflection, yoga, or other unwinding methods to encourage mental and profound prosperity.

- Restoring Way of life Decisions

- Your way of life assumes a huge part in supporting rest and recovery:

Nourishment: A reasonable eating routine wealthy in supplements and hydration upholds your body's recuperation processes.

Actual work: Standard activity adds to more readily rest quality and by and large prosperity. In any case, keep away from extraordinary exercises excessively near sleep time.

Stress The board: Foster pressure the executives procedures like using time productively, defining limits, and looking for help from companions and experts when required.

Social Associations: Keep up with significant associations with loved ones, as friendly associations offer profound help and open doors for unwinding.

- End: Re-energizing Your Life

The meaning of rest and recovery couldn't possibly be more significant. These practices are not extravagances; they are fundamental parts of a solid, satisfying life. By embracing the craft of rest and integrating recuperative practices into your way of life, you can re-energize your body, psyche, and soul.

At last, rest and recovery engage you to seek after your objectives and dreams with recharged power, making them fundamental devices for making progress and prosperity in the present requesting world.

Thus, have some time off, focus on your wellbeing, and permit yourself the reality to restore — your life will thank you for it.

Chapter 3:

1. Speedy and Compelling Cardio Exercises:

Fast and satisfying Cardio Conditioning Turbocharge Your Wellness Process In the present speedy world, sculpturing out occasion for heartiness can be a test.

Enter quick and satisfying cardio practices — your pass to turbocharging your heartiness process in not further than twinkles daily.

These exercises are complete as well as possibly successful at helping your cardiovascular good, burning calories, and keeping you in excellent condition.

Cardiovascular Pot Cardiovascular exertion is the way into a solid heart and a solid body. It builds your palpitation, further develops lung capability, and helps your body productively use oxygen.

The most amazing aspect? You do not bear hours on a routine to admit these prices. Quick and satisfying cardio conditioning can get your heart siphoning and your body perspiring right down.

violent cardio exercise(HIIT) HIIT is a cardio stalwart that's overwhelming the heartiness world. Everything revolves around short eruptions of extraordinary movement followed by brief times of rest or lower- force work out. In only 15- 20 twinkles, you can burn calories, further develop perseverance, and fabricate muscle.

This is the way to get everything rolling. Run Spans On a track or routine, run for 20- 30 seconds, also, at that point, walk or run for 10- 15 seconds. Reappraisal for 10- 15 twinkles.

Bouncing Jacks and Burpees Switch back and forth between 30 seconds of hopping jacks and 30 seconds of burpees for a full- body impact. Cycle Runs On the off chance that you approach an exercise bike, pedal as quick as possible for 30 seconds, also recoup at a further slow speed for 30 seconds.

Reappraisal for 10- 15 twinkles. Tabata Preparing Tabata is some other time- complete cardio diamond. It comprises 20 seconds of hard and fast exertion followed by 10 seconds of rest, rehashed for four twinkles(eight cycles). It's great for burning fat and working on cardiovascular heartiness.

Attempt these Tabata works out Work out with Rope Bounce as quick as possible for 20 seconds, rest for 10 seconds, and reappraisal. thickset hops do still numerous thickset hops as could be allowed for 20 seconds, also rest for 10 seconds.

trampers Connect with your center and perform trampers for 20 seconds, also recoup for 10 seconds. Bodyweight Blasters You do not inescapably in all cases need gear for a satisfying cardio exercise.

Bodyweight conditioning can get your palpitation up incontinently Burpees This full-body practice joins a thickset, push- up, and hop. do the utmost that you can in 60 seconds, also rest for 30 seconds.

Reappraisal for 10- 15 twinkles. High Knees Stand set up and run while bringing your knees as high as could really be anticipated. Do this for 30 seconds, also, at that point, recoup for 15 seconds. Reappraisal for 10- 15 twinkles.

Box Hops Track down a solid stage or step and perform box bounces for 45 seconds, traced by 15 seconds of rest. cotillion Your Direction to Wellness Who says cardio can not be amusing?

Moving is an elating and feasible system for getting your heart siphoning Zumba. Join a Zumba class or follow online educational exercises to partake in a cotillion exercise that feels like a party. hipsterism- brio Heart stimulating exercise Get your section on with high- energy hipsterism- jump cotillion schedules that join cardio and collaboration.

Line Moving Accumulates many companions and hit the cotillion bottom for an enthusiastic meeting of line moving. It's a fabulous system for mingling and exercising all the while. The Force of Fast and satisfying Cardio Conditioning

The nobility of these exercises lies in their productivity.

They can be fit into your most active days, making it nearly delicate to condemn absence of time. Indeed, indeed only 15- 20 twinkles of focused energy cardio can help your digestion, further develop your heart, and upgrade your general heartiness.

Keep in mind, prior to beginning any new work-eschewal everyday practice, it's a veterinarian to talk with a medical services professional, particularly in the event that you have any introductory medical issue.

Whenever you are cleared to go, embrace the force of quick and satisfying cardio conditioning, and watch your heartiness process turbocharge as you run, hop, and dance your direction to a better, more vivacious you.

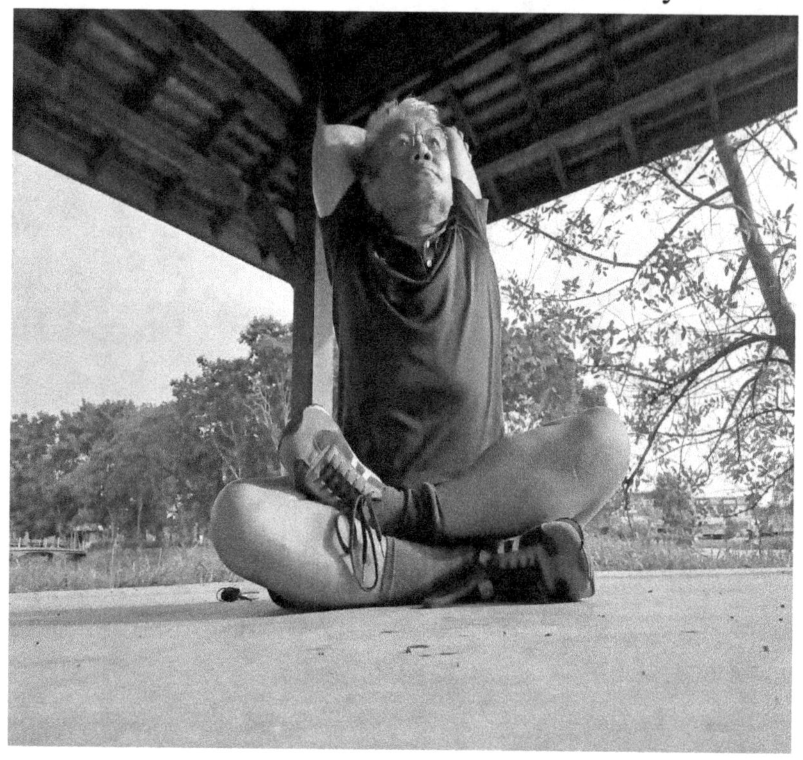

2. Kick off Your Heart: Cardiovascular Wellbeing:

Start Off Your Heart: Cardiovascular Prosperity Released

Your heart is something beyond a muscle; the motor keeps your whole body running. Embracing cardiovascular prosperity is the way into a more extended, better life. Thus, ribbon up those shoes and prepare to start off your heart with an all encompassing way to deal with cardiovascular wellbeing that is both tomfoolery and engaging.

The Main issue at hand

Your heart, that clench hand measured organ in your chest, is answerable for siphoning blood and oxygen all through your body. It's the center of your cardiovascular framework, which assumes an imperative part in your general wellbeing and prosperity. At the point when your heart is blissful, your body flourishes.

The Significance of Cardiovascular Prosperity

Cardiovascular prosperity is about something other than keeping a sound heart. It envelops the whole organization of veins, your circulatory framework, and the cycles that keep your heart solid and productive. Here's the reason it's pivotal:

Diminished Sickness Chance: A solid cardiovascular framework brings down your gamble of coronary illness, stroke, and other circulatory circumstances that can life-undermine.

Expanded Energy: When your heart is strong, it siphons oxygen-rich blood productively, furnishing your muscles and organs with the energy they need to ideally work.

Mental Lucidity: Great bloodstream upholds mental capability and can assist with forestalling conditions like dementia.

Essentialness and Life span: A solid heart adds to a functioning and satisfying life. By dealing with your cardiovascular framework, you increase your possibilities of living longer and feeling dynamic over time.

Heart-Sound Way of life Decisions

Your way of life assumes a significant part in deciding the condition of your cardiovascular prosperity. Here are a few critical propensities to embrace:

Customary Activity: Participate in normal actual work to keep your heart in top shape. Cardio exercises like energetic strolling, cycling, or swimming are amazing decisions.

Adjusted Diet: Eat an eating routine wealthy in organic products, vegetables, entire grains, lean proteins, and sound fats. Limit handled food varieties, sugar, and exorbitant salt.

Stress The executives: Track down solid ways of overseeing pressure, like care reflection, profound breathing activities, or yoga.

Sufficient Rest: Focus on rest to permit your body and heart to rest and revive.

Moderate Liquor: Assuming you drink liquor, do as such with some restraint. For some individuals, this implies one beverage each day for ladies and up to two beverages each day for men.

Sans tobacco: Abstain from smoking, and on the off chance that you smoke, look for help to stop. Smoking is a huge gambling factor for coronary illness.

The Tomfoolery Side of Cardiovascular Prosperity

Dealing with your heart doesn't need to be an errand; it very well may be a happy and empowering venture. This is the way to make it fun:

Bunch Wellness Classes: Join a neighborhood wellness class or gathering. The fellowship and shared energy can make exercises pleasant.

Dance Your Heart Out: Pursue dance classes or just dance around your lounge. Moving is a fabulous method for helping cardiovascular wellbeing while at the same time having an awesome time.

Outside Experiences: Exploit nature. Climbing, trekking, or kayaking in lovely outside settings can transform practice into an experience.

Virtual Difficulties: Take part in virtual difficulties or races. Numerous applications and sites offer fun rivalries that persuade you to move.

Sports and Games: Take part in sports you love or play fun games like badminton, tennis, or frisbee with loved ones.

Ordinary Check-Ups and Observing

Ordinary check-ups with your medical services supplier are fundamental for following your cardiovascular prosperity. These arrangements can distinguish risk factors, for example, hypertension or cholesterol, and consider early mediation.

End: Start up Your Heart

Your heart merits your consideration and care. By embracing cardiovascular prosperity, you're not simply putting resources into a more extended life; you're improving the nature of the years you have.

In this way, trim up those tennis shoes, dance to your number one tunes, and appreciate heart-quality food sources. Start off your heart,

and let it lead you to a lively, fiery, and blissful
life   where   each   thump   counts.

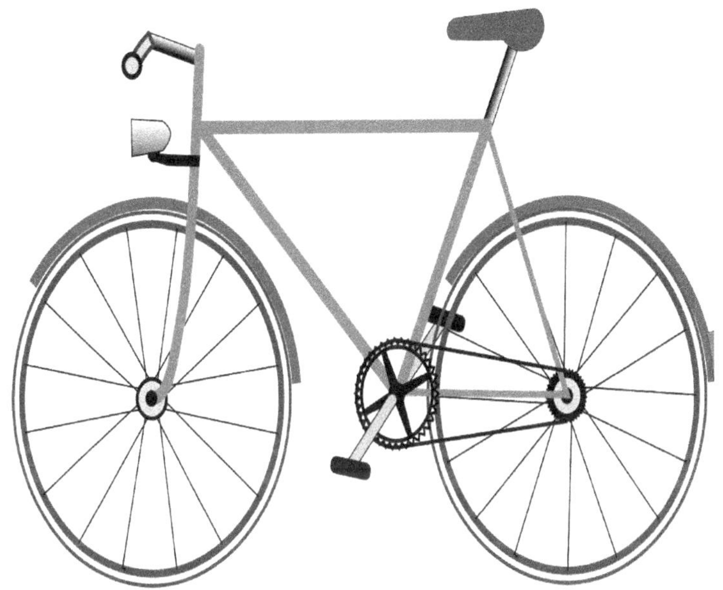

3. 5-Minute Cardio Schedules for All Wellness Levels:

5-Minute Cardio Timetables for All Wellbeing Levels: Kick off Your Wellness Process

You don't require hours at the exercise center to supercharge your wellness process. In only five minutes every day, you can raise your cardiovascular wellbeing, support your energy, and rejuvenate your prosperity. Whether you're a wellness lover or a novice, these 5-minute cardio plans take care of all wellbeing levels, guaranteeing that everybody can launch their way to a better life.

- The Force of 5-Minute Cardio

Prior to jumping into the timetables, we should investigate why 5-minute cardio meetings are unquestionably viable:

Proficiency: Five minutes is adequately short to squeeze into even the most active timetables. No more reasons about not possessing sufficient energy for workout!

Consistency: Consistency is critical to advance. A concise day to day cardio meeting is more economical than periodic longer exercises.

Jolt of energy: A fast cardio burst can strengthen you, giving a flood of energy that can endure over the course of the day.

Medical advantages: Short eruptions of cardio can work on cardiovascular wellbeing, increment digestion, and even improve state of mind.

- Amateur: Kick off Your Wellness Process

For amateurs, it's crucial to start slow and step by step. Here is a 5-minute cardio plan custom fitted to your health level:

Warm-Up (1 moment): Begin with a light run set up or energetic strolling to get your pulse up.

High Knees (1 moment): Stand set up and run while bringing your knees as high as could really be expected.

Bouncing Jacks (1 moment): Perform customary hopping jacks to lift your pulse.

Bodyweight Squats (1 moment): Do squats to connect with your leg muscles and lift your pulse.

Cool Down (1 moment): Wrap up with slow strolling or delicate extending to bring down your pulse steadily.

- Halfway Level: Lift Your Cardiovascular Wellbeing

On the off chance that a little greater power, this middle of the road 5-minute cardio plan is ideal for you:

- Warm-Up (1 moment): Begin with a light run set up or lively strolling.

Burpees (1 moment): Proceed as numerous burpees as you can in one moment. They're a full-body practice that joins squats, push-ups, and bounces.

High Knees (1 moment): Go on with high knees, however increment the force by running quicker and raising your knees higher.

Work out with Rope (1 moment): On the off chance that you have a leap rope, use it for an extreme cardiovascular exercise. On the off chance that not, imitate the movement without the rope.

Cool Down (1 moment): Get done with sluggish strolling or delicate extending to take your pulse back to typical.

- High Level: Challenge Your Cardio Cutoff points

For those looking for a heart-beating challenge, this exceptional 5-minute cardio timetable will stretch your boundaries:

- Warm-Up (1 moment): Start with a light run or lively strolling.

Run (1 moment): Run at most extreme exertion briefly. You can do this on a track, treadmill, or in an open space.

Hikers (1 moment): Perform hikers, drawing in your center and keeping your pulse high.

Box Bounces (1 moment): Track down a strong stage or step and perform box hops for 60 seconds.

Cool Down (1 moment): Get done with sluggish strolling or delicate stretching to bring down your pulse bit by bit.

Pay attention to Your Body

Regardless of your wellness level, consistently pay attention to your body. In the event that you're simply beginning or have any fundamental medical issue, talk with a medical services proficient prior to starting another work-out daily schedule. Adjust the activities depending on the situation to match your capacities and steadily increment force as your wellness moves along.

- End: Your 5-Minute Cardio Experience

With these 5-minute cardio plans, there are no more reasons for skipping exercise. No matter what your wellbeing level, these fast exercises can squeeze into your everyday daily schedule and altogether influence your cardiovascular wellbeing.

Kick off your wellness process today, and watch as five minutes daily changes your prosperity, energy levels, and generally speaking essentialness. Your heart will thank you for it!

Chapter 4:

1. Fortifying Your Center and Muscles:

Bracing Your Center and Muscles: The Way to Strength and Dependability

Your center and muscles are the unrecognized yet truly great individuals of your body, giving the establishment to strength, dependability, and generally speaking prosperity.

Bracing them isn't just about feel; it's tied in with working on your stance, forestalling wounds, and improving your day to day exercises.

Thus, we should plunge into the universe of center and muscle reinforcing to comprehend the reason why it's so critical and how you can set out on this enabling excursion.

- The Meaning of Center Strength

Your center is something beyond your abs; it incorporates a perplexing organization of muscles that settle your spine and pelvis. Here's the reason center strength matters:

Act Improvement: A solid center backings legitimate stance, decreasing the gamble of back torment and outer muscle issues.

Injury Counteraction: A steady center can forestall wounds during proactive tasks and everyday errands.

Equilibrium and Dependability: Center strength improves your equilibrium and soundness, diminishing the gamble of falls, especially as you age.

Productivity in Development: Solid center muscles make your developments more effective, from lifting objects to strolling and running.

- Muscle Strength for Day to day existence

Muscles aren't only for weight lifters; they're fundamental for everybody. Here's the reason muscle strength matters in your day to day routine:

Useful Wellness: Muscle strength empowers you to perform regular exercises easily, from conveying food to playing with your children or grandkids.

Digestion Lift: Muscles consume a bigger number of calories very still than fat. Expanding bulk can assist you with keeping a solid weight.

Bone Wellbeing: Strength preparing advances bone thickness, diminishing the gamble of osteoporosis.

Injury Strength: Solid muscles can ingest shock and safeguard your joints, decreasing the gamble of wounds.

- The Center and Muscle Fortifying Tool stash

All in all, how might you begin strengthening your center and muscles? Here are a few viable activities to remember for your everyday practice:

Boards: Boards are an incredible center activity. Stand firm on a push-up foothold with your body in an orderly fashion, drawing in your center muscles. Begin with 20-30 seconds and bit by bit increment the length.

Deadlifts: Deadlifts focus on different muscle gatherings, including your lower back, glutes, and hamstrings. Utilize legitimate structure and begin with a light weight.

Squats: Squats work your quads, hamstrings, and glutes. Perform bodyweight squats or add loads for an additional test.

Push-Ups: Push-ups are incredible for chest and rear arm muscle strength. Adjust them by doing knee push-ups if necessary.

Russian Turns: Sit on the floor, twist your knees, and recline marginally. Hold a weight or utilize a family thing like a water jug and turn your middle from one side to another to work your obliques.

Lurches: Jumps focus on your quads, hamstrings, and glutes. Perform them with legitimate structure to keep away from knee strain.

- Begin Slow and Advance Progressively

Assuming you're new to center and muscle fortifying, it's vital for start gradually and utilize appropriate structure to stay away from injury. Talk with a wellness proficient on the off chance that you're uncertain about your strategy. Start with bodyweight practices and continuously add loads or obstruction as your solidarity gets to the next level. Consistency is critical, so make these activities a customary piece of your everyday practice.

- Rest and Recuperation

Remember the significance of rest and recuperation in your reinforcing venture. Muscles need time to fix and develop further. Hold back nothing 48 hours of rest between strength instructional courses for a similar muscle bunch.

- Nourishment Matters

Nourishment assumes an essential part in muscle development and generally speaking wellbeing. Guarantee you're consuming a fair eating routine with enough protein to help muscle fix and development. Hydration is similarly urgent, as water is fundamental for muscle capability.

- End: Engage Your Body

Bracing your center and muscles isn't just about feel; it's tied in with engaging your body to have a better, more useful existence.

Solid muscles and a steady center upgrade your actual capacities, diminish the gamble of wounds, and work on your general personal satisfaction.

In this way, focus on center and muscle reinforcement in your wellness process, and watch as your body turns out to be stronger, stable, and equipped for taking on life's difficulties effortlessly.

2. Erecting a Strong root:

Bracing Your Center and Muscles The Way to Strength and Soundness Your center and muscles are the uncelebrated yet truly great individualities of your body, giving the establishment to strength, responsibility, and generally speaking substance.

Sustaining them is not just about feeling; it's tied in with working on your station, averting injuries, and perfecting your day to day exercises.

Therefore, how about we jump into the macrocosm of center and muscle buttressing to comprehend the reason why it's so vital and how you can leave on this enabling excursion.

The Meaning of Center Strength Your center is commodity beyond your abs; it incorporates a mind boggling association of muscles that balance out your chine and pelvis.

This is the reason center strength matters: Pose enhancement A solid center backings licit station, lessening the adventure of back torment and external muscle issues.

Injury Counteraction A steady center can avert injuries during visionary tasks and day to day errands.

Equilibrium and responsibility Center strength upgrades your equilibrium and security, dwindling the adventure of cascade, especially as you age.

Proficiency in Development Solid center muscles make your developments more complete, from lifting objects to tromping and running.

Muscle Strength for Day to day actuality Muscles are not only for weight lifters; they are abecedarian for everybody.

This is the reason muscle strength matters in your regular routine Useful Wellness Muscle strength empowers you to perform regular exercises fluently, from conveying food to playing with your children or grandkids. Digestion Lift Muscles consume a lesser number of calories veritably still than fat.

Expanding bulk can help you with keeping a sound weight. Bone Good Strength preparing advances bone consistency, dwindling the adventure of osteoporosis.

Injury Versatility Solid muscles can assimilate shock and guard your joints, lessening the adventure of injuries.

The Center and Muscle Fortifying Tool store All by each, how might you begin strengthening your center and muscles?

Then are many important conditioning to flash back for your everyday practice Boards Boards are an inconceivable center exertion.

Stand establishment on a drive- up footing with your body in an orderly fashion, drawing in your center muscles. Begin with 20- 30 seconds and steadily proliferation the span.

Deadlifts concentrate on different muscle gatherings, including your lower back, glutes, and hamstrings.

use licit structure and begin with a light weight. Squats Squats work your closes, hamstrings, and glutes. Perform bodyweight syllables or add loads for a fresh test.

Push- Ups Push- ups are phenomenal for caskets and hinder arm muscle strength. Acclimate them by doing knee drive- ups if necessary.

Russian Turns: Sit on the bottom, twist your knees, and slope hard. Hold a weight or use a family thing like a water flagon and curve your middle from one side to another to work your obliques.

Rushes Thrusts focus on your closes, hamstrings, and glutes.

Perform them with applicable structure to stay down from knee strain.

Begin Slow and Advance Step by step Assuming you are new to center and muscle fortifying, it's a veterinarian for launching gradually and using licit structure to keep down from injury.

Talk with a heartiness complete on the off chance that you are uncertain about your procedure.

Start with bodyweight practices and continuously add loads or opposition as your solidarity gets to the coming position.

thickness is critical, so make these conditioning a standard piece of your diurnal schedule.

Rest and Recuperation Flash back the significance of rest and rehabilitation in your fortifying excursion.

Muscles need time to fix and develop farther. Hold back nothing 48 hours of rest between strength educational meetings for an analogous muscle bunch.

Aliment Matters Aliment assumes a pivotal part in muscle development and in general good.

Guarantee you are consuming a reasonable eating routine with enough protein to help muscle fix and development.

Hydration is also critical, as water is a vector for muscle capability.

End Engage Your Body Amping your center and muscles is not just about style; it's tied in with enabling your body to have a better, more useful actuality.

Solid muscles and a steady center upgrade your factual capacities, dwindle the adventure of injuries, and work on your general particular satisfaction.

Therefore, concentrate on center and muscle buttressing in your heartiness process, and watch as your body turns out to be stronger, stable, and equipped for taking on life's difficulties painlessly.

3. Absolute Body Exertion in Only 5 twinkles:

Outright Body Molding in Just 5 Twinkles The Force of Fast and Successful Exercises In our speedy lives, sculpturing our occasion for exercise can be a test, still imagine a script in which you could negotiate outright body molding in only 5 twinkles.

It might sound unrealistic, yet with the right conditioning and force, you can change your body and lift your heartiness in a short time. We should probe the idea of super effective exercises and how they can help you with negotiating striking issues in only a couple of moments daily.

The Sorcery of Extreme cardio exercise(HIIT) The riddle behind outright body molding in a short time lies in a heartiness peculiarity known as Extreme cardio exercise, or HIIT. HIIT is an exercise fashion that consolidates short explosions of focused energy practice with brief times of rest or lower- power action.

This approach is intended to boost calorie consumption, proliferation digestion, and work on general heartiness in a negligible measure of time. This is the reason HIIT is so successful. Effective Calorie Consume HIIT exercises light a critical number of calories in a brief time frame, making them ideal for weight reduction and fat consuming.

Supported Digestion HIIT can lift your digestion, making your body consume calories indeed after the exercise is further than, a peculiarity known as the" afterburn" impact. Effective HIIT exercises are extraordinarily time-productive.

You can finish a full- body exercise in only a couple of moments, making it simple to squeeze into a bustling schedule. Working on Cardiovascular Wellbeing HIIT can upgrade your heart well by expanding cardiovascular heartiness and bringing down palpitation.

Muscle Protection Anyhow of their brief term, HIIT exercises can help save and indeed form with inclining bulk.

A 5- Minute HIIT Routine for Outright Body Molding Presently, we should jump into an illustration 5- nanosecond HIIT schedule that can help you with negotiating outright body molding Warm- Up(1 moment) Begin with light running set up or bouncing jacks to get your palpitation up and set up your muscles for the exercise. thickset hops(30 seconds) Perform thickset hops, where you hunker down and violently hop up, landing delicately with bowed knees.

Push- Ups(30 seconds) Drop to the ground and do as numerous drive- ups as you can with licit structure. Acclimate by doing knee drive- ups if necessary. trampers(30 seconds) Get into a board position and cover getting your knees toward your casket for a running movement.

High Knees(30 seconds) Stand set up and run while bringing your knees as high as conceivable with each step. Cool Down(1 moment) Get done with sluggish tromping or delicate extending to bring down your palpitation sluggishly.

Tips
Variety Change up the conditioning and power to keep your body drawn in and forestall situations. food and Recuperation For outright body molding, supplementing your exercises with a reasonable eating routine and satisfactory recovery is vital food Energy your body with an indeed eating authority that incorporates different supplements.

Protein is a vector for muscle fix and development. Hydration remains veritably important doused , as water is essential for muscle capability and rehabilitation. Rest Permit your body time to recoup and fix. Guarantee you are getting sufficient rest and integrating rest days into your everyday practice.

Integrate HIIT into Your Way of life The excellence of HIIT is its inflexibility and versatility. You can redo your HIIT routine to accommodate your heartiness position, objects, and accessible time. Whether you are an exertion sucker hoping to expand your issues or a rookie looking for a productive system for beginning your heartiness process, HIIT can be customized to your needs.

End Accomplish Outright Body Molding While a 5- nanosecond HIIT exercise may not displant longer, further thorough heartiness schedules fully, it tends to be a distinct advantage for those occasions when time is confined. The way to progress is thickness and propelling yourself during those short explosions of serious exertion.

By integrating HIIT into your way of life, you can negotiate outright body molding, help your heartiness, and witness the fantastic advantages of extreme cardio exercise in only a couple of moments daily.

Therefore, prepare to start to perspire and open your body's maximum capacity with this time-effective and strong exercise procedure.

Outright Body Molding in Just 5 Minutes: The Force of Fast and Successful Exercises

In our speedy lives, carving out opportunities for exercise can be a test, however imagine a scenario in which you could accomplish outright body molding in only 5 minutes.

It might sound unrealistic, yet with the right activities and force, you can change your body and lift your wellness in a short time. We should investigate the idea of super effective exercises and how they can assist you with accomplishing striking outcomes in only a couple of moments daily.

- The Sorcery of Extreme cardio exercise (HIIT)

The mystery behind outright body molding in a short time lies in a wellness peculiarity known as Extreme cardio exercise, or HIIT. HIIT is an exercise technique that consolidates short explosions of focused energy practice with brief times of rest or lower-power action. This approach is intended to boost calorie consumption, increment digestion, and work on general wellness in a negligible measure of time.

- Here's the reason HIIT is so successful:

Effective Calorie Consume: HIIT exercises light a critical number of calories in a brief time frame, making them ideal for weight reduction and fat consuming.

Supported Digestion: HIIT can lift your digestion, making your body consume calories even after the exercise is more than, a peculiarity known as the "afterburn" impact.

Efficient: HIIT exercises are extraordinarily time-productive. You can finish a full-body exercise in only a couple of moments, making it simple to squeeze into a bustling timetable.

Worked on Cardiovascular Wellbeing: HIIT can upgrade your heart wellbeing by expanding cardiovascular wellness and bringing down pulse.

Muscle Protection: Regardless of their brief term, HIIT exercises can assist save and even form with inclining bulk.

Outright Body Molding in Just 5 twinkles

The Force of Fast and Successful Exercises In our speedy lives, sculpturing our occasion for exercise can be a test, still imagine a script in which you could negotiate outright body molding in only 5 twinkles.

It might sound unrealistic, yet with the right conditioning and force, you can change your body and lift your heartiness in a short time.

We should probe the idea of super effective exercises and how they can help you with negotiating striking issues in only a couple of moments daily.

The Sorcery of Extreme cardio exercise(HIIT) The riddle behind outright body molding in a short time lies in a heartiness peculiarity known as Extreme cardio exercise, or HIIT.

HIIT is an exercise fashion that consolidates short explosions of focused energy practice with brief times of rest or lower- power action.

This approach is intended to boost calorie consumption, proliferation digestion, and work on in general heartiness in a negligible measure of time.

This is the reason HIIT is so successful. Effective Calorie Consume HIIT exercises light a critical number of calories in a brief time frame, making them ideal for weight reduction and fat consuming.

Supported Digestion HIIT can lift your digestion, making your body consume calories indeed after the exercise is further than, a peculiarity known as the" afterburn" impact. Effective HIIT exercises are extraordinarily time-productive.

You can finish a full- body exercise in only a couple of moments, making it simple to squeeze into a bustling schedule.

Working on Cardiovascular Wellbeing HIIT can upgrade your heart well by expanding cardiovascular heartiness and bringing down palpitation.

Muscle Protection Anyhow of their brief term, HIIT exercises can help save and indeed form with inclining bulk. A 5- Minute HIIT Routine for Outright Body Molding Presently, we should jump into an illustration 5- nanosecond HIIT schedule that can help you with negotiating outright body molding Warm- Up(1 moment) Begin with light running set up or bouncing jacks to get your palpitation up and set up your muscles for the exercise.

thickset hops(30 seconds) Perform thickset hops, where you hunker down and violently hop up, landing delicately with bowed knees.

Push- Ups(30 seconds) Drop to the ground and do as numerous drive- ups as you can with licit structure. Acclimate by doing knee drive- ups if necessary.

trampers(30 seconds) Get into a board position and cover getting your knees toward your casket for a running movement.

High Knees(30 seconds) Stand set up and run while bringing your knees as high as conceivable with each step.

Cool Down(1 moment) Get done with sluggish tromping or delicate extending to bring down your palpitation sluggishly.

Tips for Progress To take full advantage of your 5- nanosecond HIIT exercise Power Matters Stretch yourself to the edge during the extreme focus spans.

You ought to feel tested, yet good ought to constantly start effects out. licit Structure Guarantee you are involving the right structure for each exertion to forestall injuries.

While a solitary 5- nanosecond meeting can be successful, integrating HIIT exercises into your schedule many times each week will yield better results over the long haul.

Variety Change up the conditioning and power to keep your body drawn in and forestall situations.

food and Recuperation For outright body molding, supplementing your exercises with a reasonable eating routine and satisfactory recovery is vital food Energy your body with an indeed eating authority that incorporates different supplements.

Protein is a vector for muscle fix and development. Hydration remains veritably important doused , as water is essential for muscle capability and rehabilitation.

Rest Permit your body time to recoup and fix. Guarantee you are getting sufficient rest and integrating rest days into your everyday practice.

Integrate HIIT into Your Way of life The excellence of HIIT is its inflexibility and versatility.

You can redo your HIIT routine to accommodate your heartiness position, objects, and accessible time.

Whether you are an exertion sucker hoping to expand your issues or a rookie looking for a productive system for beginning your heartiness process, HIIT can be customized to your needs.

End Accomplish Outright Body Molding While a 5- nanosecond HIIT exercise may not displant longer, further thorough heartiness schedules fully, it tends to be a distinct advantage for those occasions when time is confined.

The way to progress is thickness and propelling yourself during those short explosions of serious exertion.

By integrating HIIT into your way of life, you can negotiate outright body molding, help your heartiness, and witness the fantastic advantages of extreme cardio exercise in only a couple of moments daily.

Therefore, prepare to start to perspire and open your body's maximum capacity with this time-effective and strong exercise procedure.

Chapter 5:

1. Adaptability and Portability:

Flexibility and Conveyability: The Powerful Couple of Current Living

In the present quick moving world, the capacity to adjust and stay versatile isn't simply profitable; it's fundamental for progress and prosperity. These two characteristics, flexibility and conveyability, structure a unique pair that enables us to explore life's difficulties, quickly jump all over chances, and make every second count.

- Versatility: The Specialty of Flourishing in Change

Versatility is the ability of embracing change with great enthusiasm, acclimating to new conditions, and flourishing in the midst of vulnerability. Here's the reason flexibility is significant:

Strength: Versatility cultivates flexibility, assisting us with returning from difficulties, adapt to misfortune, and arise more grounded.

Advancement: It drives development by empowering us to think inventively, investigate new arrangements, and rock the boat.

Development: Versatile people are bound to embrace self-awareness and advancement, persistently endeavoring to work on themselves.

Improved Connections: Adaptability in adjusting to others' necessities and viewpoints prompts more hearty and agreeable connections.

Professional success: In the expert domain, flexibility is a profoundly sought-after ability, permitting people to succeed in quickly evolving ventures.

- Compactness: Opportunity to Move and Develop

Conveyability alludes to our ability to stay spry and adaptable, liberated from troubles that could prevent our portability. Here's the reason transportability is priceless:

Opportunity: It awards us the opportunity to investigate new open doors, travel to new spots, and make the most of life's undertakings.

Moderation: Versatility supports a moderate way of life, underlining encounters over belongings and decreasing mess in our lives.

Asset Productivity: Convenient innovation and instruments advance asset effectiveness, empowering us to work, interface, and engage ourselves in a hurry.

Balance between serious and fun activities: It considers a better balance between fun and serious activities by empowering us to take our work with us, breaking liberated from the imperatives of a conventional office.

Ecological Effect: Conveyability frequently implies decreased driving and a more modest natural impression, lining up with manageability objectives.

- The Convergence of Flexibility and Compactness
- These two characteristics are entwined, each upgrading the other's effect:

Adaptability in Way of life: Embracing flexibility permits us to fit our way of life to evolving conditions. Being convenient means we can do as such without being fastened to a particular area.

Vocation Development: In a quickly developing position market, flexibility empowers us to turn our professions. Conveyability guarantees we can take those new abilities and open doors any place they lead.

Mechanical Strengthening: Versatile innovation upholds flexibility by empowering remote work, learning, and correspondence, making it more straightforward than at any other time to adjust to developing circumstances.

Worldwide Citizenship: The capacity to adjust to different societies and conditions, combined with the opportunity to travel, makes worldwide residents who can flourish in an interconnected world.

Wellbeing and Health: Both versatility and movability are fundamental for keeping up with physical and mental prosperity, permitting us to track down the right equilibrium throughout everyday life.

- Embracing Flexibility and Conveyability
- To outfit the capability of versatility and transportability completely:

Receptiveness: Develop a receptive outlook and a readiness to embrace change as a chance for development.

Deep rooted Learning: Constantly put resources into mastering and getting new abilities to remain versatile in an impacting world.

Smooth out Belongings: Clean up and focus on encounters and fundamentals over material belongings.

Remote Work: If conceivable, investigate remote work choices, which offer both versatility and compactness.

Adjusted Living: Take a stab at a healthy lifestyle that incorporates work, self-awareness, and relaxation, all while being versatile to developing conditions.

- End: Flourishing in a Consistently Impacting World

In the advanced age, versatility and conveyability are not simply helpful characteristics; they are fundamental for individual and expert achievement.

By embracing change, remaining spry, and using versatile assets, we can explore the intricacies of our steadily impacting world with certainty and force.

These unique characteristics engage us to lead advancing lives loaded up with undertakings, development, and the opportunity to pursue our fantasies, unburdened by the requirements of the past.

Thus, adjust and stay compact, and let these characteristics be your compass in the excursion of life.

2. The Way to Remaining Lithe:

The Best approach to Staying Agile: Embrace Adaptability for a Dynamic Life

In a world that is continually moving, staying flexible - both in body and brain - is the way to embrace the difficulties and open doors life presents. Agile, significance, graceful, adaptable, and coordinated, is a quality that goes past actual wellness. It incorporates flexibility, versatility, and a receptive way to deal with life. In this way, how about we investigate the way to staying agile and energetic, regardless of your age or conditions.

- Physical Agile: Adaptability for Your Body

Physical agile is tied in with keeping your body, areas of strength for adaptable, though. Here's the reason it's urgent:

Joint Wellbeing: Adaptability practices assist with keeping up with solid joints, decreasing the gamble of wounds and joint-related issues.

- Pose: Great stance depends on adaptability and strength in the muscles that help your spine.

Injury Avoidance: Adaptable muscles are less inclined to strain and injury, making flexibility a fundamental part of a functioning way of life.

Improved Scope of Movement: Being flexible permits you to move all the more openly, whether it's arriving at high retirement, playing sports, or appreciating side interests.

Stress Decrease: Extending and adaptability activities can lessen muscle pressure and advance unwinding, prompting work on mental prosperity.

- To embrace physical agile:

Integrate extending practices into your day to day daily schedule.
Investigate exercises like yoga or Pilates that upgrade adaptability and strength.
Focus on legitimate warm-ups and cooldowns when proactive tasks.
Mental Agile: Adaptability of the Psyche

- Mental flexibility is tied in with supporting an open and versatile attitude. It includes:

- Flexibility: Being available to change and ready to conform to new conditions and difficulties.

- Inventiveness: Developing an imaginative and creative way to deal with critical thinking.
- Close to home Flexibility: Creating profound solidarity to adapt to life's highs and lows.
- Liberality: Being responsive to novel thoughts, points of view, and encounters.
- Stress The executives: Figuring out how to oversee pressure through care and unwinding strategies.
- To develop mental flexible:

Practice care contemplation to upgrade profound strength and stress the board.

Take part in deep rooted figuring out how to keep your psyche spry and open to novel thoughts.

Search out assorted points of view and participate in conversations with individuals who have various perspectives.

Way of life Flexible: Difficult exercise in Current Living

Way of life includes finding some kind of harmony between different parts of life to keep up with prosperity. This is the way it adds to a lively life:

Balance between serious and fun activities: Focusing on private time, connections, and relaxation close by proficient obligations.

Manageable Living: Embracing eco-accommodating practices and consuming carefully to diminish the natural effect.

Social Associations: Sustaining significant associations with family, companions, and the local area.

Experience and Investigation: Embracing new encounters, travel, and side interests to keep life invigorating.

Taking care of oneself: Setting aside some margin for taking care of oneself exercises that advance physical and psychological well-being.

- To lead a way of life flexible:

Put down stopping points to safeguard your own time and prosperity.
Integrate economical practices into your everyday existence, like lessening waste and rationing energy.

Effectively put resources into building and keeping up with social associations.
The Flexible Excursion: A Long lasting Pursuit

Staying flexible isn't an objective yet a deep rooted venture. It requires a pledge to ordinary actual work, progressing mentally and close to home development, and a decent way to deal with life.

As you embrace adaptability in body, brain, and way of life, you'll find that it's the way to living an energetic, satisfying life, no matter what your age or conditions.

Thus, leave on the way to staying agile, and let adaptability and flexibility be your aides as you explore the exciting bends in the road of life's excursion.

Embrace the difficulties, jump all over the chances, and enjoy the experiences of euphoria and development en route.

3. Extending and Versatility Activities for 40+:

Extending and Versatility Conditioning for 40 Broadening and Rigidity Exercises for 40 Embrace Imperativeness at Each Stage As we progress, keeping up with rigidity and inflexibility turns out to be precipitously significant for generally substance and particular satisfaction.

Embracing exercises that emphasis on broadening and rigidity can help with keeping you dynamic, dynamic, and prepared to handle life's guests , indeed in your 40s and also some.

Then is the reason these exercises matter and an affable way of integrating them into your diurnal practice.

The Significance of Broadening and Rigidity common Good Broadening practices help with keeping your joints flexible and lessen the adventure of firmness and torture that can accompany age.

Equilibrium and Security Inflexibility exercises challenge your equilibrium and reliableness, lessening the adventure of cascade and injuries. Afflict Counteraction Standard extending can alleviate muscle pressure and forestall normal palpitating painfulness.

Upgraded compass of Movement Rigidity practices work on your compass of movement, making day to day exercises simpler and further agreeable. Mental Unwinding Broadening and inflexibility exercises constantly integrate care and unwinding styles, helping your cerebral substance.

Fun Exercises for Expanding and Adaptability Yoga Yoga is a fabulous practice that joins extending, equilibrium, and care. There are different styles to suit your inclinations, from delicate Hatha yoga to seriously testing Vinyasa or Power yoga. Pilates Pilates centers around center strength, rigidity, and equilibrium.

It's a brilliant system for conditioning muscles and upgrading generally speaking body awareness. Yoga This antiquated Chinese practice advances equilibrium, rigidity, and internal unwinding through sluggish, streaming developments. Yoga is particularly useful for further developing equilibrium and soundness. cotillion Moving is a great system for further developing rigidity and collaboration. Consider taking cotillion classes like artful cotillion , salsa, or tango, or principally dance to your number one music in the solace of your home.

Planting Cultivating includes numerous developments that can ameliorate your rigidity and strength. It's a down to earth system for partaking in the outside and remaining dynamic. Extending Schedule Plan a day to day extending schedule that objects significant muscle gatherings.

This should be possible in the first part of the day or before bed and requires a couple of moments. Swimming Swimming is a low-influence practice that gives an inconceivable full- body exercise.

The lightness of water makes it ideal for delicate extending and expanding rigidity. Consolidating Broadening and Rigidity into Day to day actuality Remain Reliable Devote a particular time every day or week to your picked expanding and inflexibility exercises. thickness is vital to encountering the advantages. Stir It Up multifariousness is vital for keeping effects fascinating.

Attempt colorful exercises to forestall fatigue and work different muscle gatherings. Warm-Up and Chill Off In every case warm up previous to extending or sharing in inflexibility exercises, and finish up with a cool-down period to grease your muscles. Stand by harkening to Your Body Focus on your body's signs. In the event that you feel torture or agony during a movement, change or stop to forestall injury.

Careful Practice Integrate care into your diurnal schedule. Center around your breath and sensations during extending or yoga to upgrade unwinding. Decision A Deep confirmed Excursion of Imperativeness Expanding and rigidity exercises aren't just about factual rigidity; they are tied in with embracing essentialness at each phase of life.

By making these exercises a piece of your diurnal practice, you can further develop your factual substance, internal unwinding, and generally speaking particular satisfaction in your 40s and also some. Recollect that it's noway beyond any good time to begin or do with these practices.

Whether you are a precisely prepared yogi or a total rookie, there are exercises and schedules reasonable for everybody. Therefore, set out on this excursion of essentialness and recommend the magnificent liability that broadening and inflexibility exercises offer for a satisfying, dynamic, and lively life.

Chapter 6:

1. Careful Development and Stress Decrease:

Cautious Turn of events and Stress Abatement: The Amicable Way to Prosperity

In the buzzing about current life, the quest for self-awareness frequently becomes the overwhelming focus. However, similarly significant is the craft of pressure decrease, which supplements cautious advancement delightfully. Together, they make an agreeable way to deal with prosperity that enables people to flourish in all parts of life. We should investigate the cooperative energy between cautious turn of events and stress decrease and how it can prompt a seriously satisfying and adjusted presence.

The Cautious Advancement Excursion

Cautious advancement is the purposeful and insightful course of improving one's abilities, information, and generally speaking self-awareness. It's tied in with putting forth clear objectives, persistently learning, and pursuing turning into one's best self. Here's the reason it's fundamental:

Persistent Improvement: Cautious improvement encourages a mentality of deep rooted learning and improvement, permitting people to adjust to new difficulties and potential open doors.

Expanded Confidence: As you accomplish your advancement objectives, your confidence and self-assurance develop, decidedly affecting your psychological prosperity.

Professional success: Further developed abilities and information open ways to new vocation potential open doors and expert development.

Improved Critical thinking: Cautious advancement outfits people with the devices to tackle complex issues and pursue informed choices.

The Pressure Decrease Workmanship

Stress decrease is the act of overseeing and reducing pressure to advance mental and actual wellbeing. It's an essential part of prosperity on the grounds that:

Mental Lucidity: Diminishing pressure improves mental lucidity, empowering people to think all the more obviously and settle on better choices.

Close to home Equilibrium: Stress decreases methods like care and contemplation advance profound equilibrium and flexibility, diminishing the gamble of uneasiness and despondency.

Worked on Actual Wellbeing: Bringing down feelings of anxiety can emphatically affect actual wellbeing, diminishing the gamble of coronary illness, hypertension, and other pressure related conditions.

Better Connections: Decreased pressure prompts worked on relational connections, as people are more understanding, compassionate, and responsive.

The Cooperative energy of Cautious Turn of events and Stress Decrease

While cautious turn of events and stress decrease are important exclusively, their collaboration can make a significant effect on by and large prosperity. This is the way they complete one another:

Stress Decrease Supports Learning: A quiet and peaceful brain is more responsive to learning and self-improvement. Stress decrease strategies like reflection can improve concentration and focus.

Cautious Improvement Upgrades Versatility: Growing new abilities and information can increment strength, assisting individuals with better adapting to upsetting circumstances.

Adjusted Way to deal with Objectives: Cautious advancement permits people to define and seek after significant objectives, while stress decrease deals with the nervousness and tension that can accompany desire.

Comprehensive Wellbeing: The mix of cautious turn of events and stress decrease tends to both mental and actual prosperity, bringing about an all encompassing way to deal with wellbeing.

Expanded Imagination: Stress decrease practices can invigorate inventiveness, upgrading critical abilities to think and creative reasoning.

Integrating Cautious Turn of events and Stress Decrease into Day to day existence

Care Reflection: Begin your day with a short care contemplation meeting to diminish pressure and advance mental lucidity.

Objective Setting: Lay out clear and reachable improvement objectives, both actually and expertly, and pursue them deliberately.

Normal Activity: Participate in customary actual work to deliver pressure diminishing endorphins and keep up with in general wellbeing.

Good dieting: A fair eating regimen wealthy in supplements can uphold both cautious turn of events and stress decrease.

Using time productively: Effective using time effectively can diminish pressure by guaranteeing you possess devoted energy for personal growth and unwinding.

Decision: An Amicable Excursion to Prosperity

In the journey for self-awareness and prosperity, the agreeable combination of cautious turn of events and stress decrease is a strong methodology.

It enables people to accomplish their objectives while keeping up with mental and actual wellbeing, versatility, and a fair point of view on life's difficulties.

Embrace this collaboration, and you'll wind up on a satisfying excursion towards a more enhanced and agreeable presence.

2. The Psyche Body Association:

The Mind Body Affiliation: Supporting the Brain Body Association for All encompassing Prosperity

The perplexing connection between the brain and the body is a significant and frequently misjudged force that can fundamentally influence our general prosperity. This collaboration, known as the mind body affiliation, features the significant impact of our viewpoints, feelings, and mental state on our actual wellbeing as well as the other way around. We should investigate the force of this association and how supporting it can prompt comprehensive prosperity.

- Understanding the Mind Body Affiliation

The mind body affiliation is the significant association between our psychological and profound state (mind) and our actual wellbeing and working (body). This perplexing association isn't just clear in what our feelings can mean for our actual wellbeing yet in addition in what actual wellbeing can mean for our psychological and profound prosperity.

- The Force of Positive Feelings on Wellbeing

Stress Decreases: Positive feelings like happiness, appreciation, and adore can diminish feelings of anxiety. Lower pressure is related to working on cardiovascular wellbeing, lower irritation, and improved invulnerable capability.

Torment The board: An uplifting perspective can further develop torment resistance and diminish the view of torment. To this end giggling is in many cases named the best medication.

Life span: Studies propose that people with a more uplifting perspective on life will quite often live longer and appreciate better generally speaking wellbeing.

Strength: Positive feelings upgrade versatility, assisting people with returning from difficulty all the more successfully.

- The Effect of Gloomy Feelings on Wellbeing

Persistent Pressure: Delayed pressure or pessimistic feelings can prompt ongoing pressure, which is connected to a scope of medical problems, including coronary illness, heftiness, and psychological well-being problems.

Irritation: Gloomy feelings can set off aggravation in the body, adding to different medical conditions.

Safe Capability: Constant pessimistic feelings can debilitate the invulnerable framework, making people more helpless to disease.

Psychological well-being: Pessimistic feelings can worsen emotional well-being conditions like nervousness and sorrow.

- The Body's Effect on the Brain

Exercise and Temperament: Active work discharges endorphins, which are regular mind-set lifters. Customary activity is connected to decreased side effects of sadness and nervousness.

Sustenance: A reasonable eating regimen with fundamental supplements can uphold mind wellbeing and mental capability, impacting temperament and mental prosperity.

Rest: Quality rest is essential for emotional well-being and mental capability. Rest unsettling influences can add to state of mind issues.

Stomach Mind Association: Arising research recommends areas of strength for a between stomach wellbeing and psychological well-being. A sound stomach microbiome can decidedly influence temperament and comprehension.

- Supporting the Mind Body Relationship for Comprehensive Prosperity

Care and Reflection: These practices can assist you with turning out to be more mindful of your viewpoints and feelings, permitting you to decidedly oversee and divert them.

Actual work: Participating in ordinary activity helps your actual wellbeing as well as significantly affects your psychological and close to home prosperity.

Nourishment: A reasonable eating routine wealthy in organic products, vegetables, entire grains, and incline proteins can uphold both physical and psychological well-being.

Stress Decrease Methods: Integrate pressure decrease rehearses like profound breathing activities, moderate muscle unwinding, and yoga into your everyday practice.

- Quality Rest: Focus on rest cleanliness practices to guarantee peaceful and helpful rest.

Look for Help: In the event that you're battling with psychological well-being issues or persistent gloomy feelings, make it a point to get help from a specialist or guide.

- The Excursion to Comprehensive Prosperity

Supporting the mind body affiliation is an excursion that requires continuous responsibility and mindfulness. It includes settling on cognizant decisions to focus on mental and close to home well being close to actual prosperity. Here are a few extra tips to cultivate this association:

Practice Appreciation: Develop a propensity for appreciation by routinely considering the positive parts of your life.

Cultivate Positive Connections: Encircle yourself with strong, positive people who elevate and energize you.

Limit Negative Sources of info: Be aware of the substance you consume, including news and web-based entertainment. Limit openness to pessimism whenever the situation allows.

Participate in Imaginative Exercises: Inventive outlets like workmanship, music, or composing can be remedial and advance positive feelings.

Remain Inquisitive: Embrace interest and deep rooted figuring out how to keep your brain dynamic and locked in.

- End: Embrace the Force of the Mind Body Affiliation

The mind-body affiliation is a strong power that can either move us towards all encompassing prosperity or drag us down into a pattern of pressure and pessimism.

By recognizing and supporting this association, we can enable ourselves to have better, more adjusted existences.

As you set out on this excursion of comprehensive prosperity, recollect that each curtain idea, sound decision, and demonstration of taking care of oneself adds to an amicable mind-body relationship that prompts a seriously satisfying and lively presence.

3. Speedy Unwinding Procedures for a Bustling Life:

133

Expedient Loosening up Techniques for a Clamoring Life: Tracking down Quiet in the Confusion

In the present speedy world, where furious timetables and unending daily agendas frequently rule our lives, finding snapshots of harmony and unwinding becomes principal. Expedient loosening techniques offer a relief from the confusion, permitting us to quickly restore our psyches and bodies. We should dig into a few successful procedures to assist you with tracking down quiet in the midst of the buzzing about day to day existence.

- The Requirement for Fast Loosening up

In the hurricane of present day life, it's not difficult to become involved with the rush and disregard the significance of unwinding and loosening up. In any case, these short rests are fundamental because of multiple factors:

Stress Decrease: Speedy loosening up procedures can assist with diminishing feelings of anxiety, improving mental and profound prosperity.

Further developed Concentration: Enjoying short reprieves to loosen up can support fixation and efficiency, permitting you to actually handle assignments more.

Upgraded Inventiveness: Snapshots of unwinding can start imagination and creative reasoning, helping both individual and expert life.

Actual Wellbeing: Fast loosening up can decidedly affect actual wellbeing by diminishing strain and advancing unwinding.

- Fast Loosening up Methodology to Attempt

Profound Relaxing: Require a couple of moments to zero in on your breath. Breathe in profoundly through your nose, permitting your mid-region to rise, and afterward breathe out leisurely through your mouth. Profound breathing can rapidly quiet the sensory system and decrease pressure.

Smaller than expected Reflection: Track down a peaceful space, shut your eyes, and focus on your breath or a quieting word or expression. Indeed, even a short reflection meeting can give a feeling of quiet and clearness.

Stretch Breaks: Stand up and extend your body for a couple of moments. Center around delivering strain in your neck, shoulders, and back. Extending can reduce actual pressure and advance unwinding.

Nature Association: Put in no time flat outside if conceivable. Whether it's a stroll in the park, a second on your overhang, or essentially looking at the sky, interfacing with nature can extraordinarily calm.

Careful Eating: When you eat, be completely present and enjoy each nibble. This act of careful eating feeds your body as well as gives a psychological break.

Moderate Muscle Unwinding: Tense and afterward discharge each muscle bunch in your body, beginning from your toes and moving gradually up to your head. This procedure can rapidly ease actual strain.

Positive Perception: Shut your eyes and picture a quiet and peaceful spot. Envision yourself there, connecting every one of your faculties. Perception can move your psyche to a serene state.

Integrating Rapid Loosening up into Your Daily schedule

Plan Breaks: Allot brief breaks over the course of your day to integrate speedy loosening up methods. This can be basically as straightforward as requiring a couple of moments between gatherings or errands.

Make Ceremonies: Create loosening up customs that signal the finish of a bustling period and the start of unwinding. It very well may be pretty much as direct as making some home grown tea or participating shortly in profound relaxing.

Limit Screen Time: Decrease screen time, particularly before sleep time. The blue light discharged by screens can upset rest designs. Utilize this time for fast loosening up systems all things considered.

Practice Appreciation: Put shortly every day pondering what you're thankful for. This positive outlook shift can add to a feeling of satisfaction and unwinding.

Put down Stopping points: Lay out limits to safeguard your unwinding time. Impart your requirements to companions, family, or associates, so they grasp the significance of these minutes.

- The Force of Expedient Loosening up Systems

Fast loosening up systems are like smaller than normal resets for your brain and body, permitting you to explore the bedlam of existence effortlessly. They give snapshots of peacefulness that can be both reviving and fortifying, guaranteeing you stay adjusted and centered in the midst of the hecticness.

Also, these methods engage you to recapture command over your profound state, diminish pressure, and upgrade your general prosperity. Integrating them into your day to day schedule can prompt a more loose and versatile you.

All in all, finding quiet in the mayhem of a clamoring life isn't just feasible yet in addition fundamental for your psychological, profound, and actual wellbeing.

Rapid loosening up strategies offer a viable and successful means to accomplish this equilibrium, permitting you to enjoy the experiences of serenity in your bustling world.

Thus, embrace these procedures, and allow them to be your asylum of quiet in the midst of the hurricane of present day life.

Chapter 7:

1. Following Advancement and Remaining Propelled:

Following Headway and Remaining Moved Following Development and Staying Affected The Specialty of Determined Headway Life is a journey of steady turn of events and upgrade, and to finance on it, we ought to follow movement persistently and remain ceaselessly pushed.

This exceptional two or three advancement and mitigation can push us toward our items and dreams with terrible affirmation. We ought to test the cooperation between these two thoughts and how they can incite a reality of horrid progression.

The Journey for Movement isn't just about showing up at the ideal; it's about the trip of interminable improvement, education, and advancement.

Then, at that point, is the explanation it's so basic tone-care Advance supports tone-care, allowing individuals to track down their actual limit and continually advance.

Achievement of items the fundamental inspiration draws you closer to your articles and dreams, drowsily and designedly.

Flexibility Movement further develops firmness, enabling individuals to thrive in a continually affecting world.

Improvement Pursuing development upholds innovative rationale and decisive reasoning, which are abecedarian for progress.

The Power of Lightning Easing is the energy that keeps us pushing ahead, regardless, when hardships crop .

Then, at that point, the explanation easing expects a huge part Drive and Confirmation Motivation stimulates the drive and affirmation expected to dominate obstacles and progress forward.

Focus It stays aware of revolving around your articles and monitors interferences. Flexibility Lightening collects strength, allowing individuals to return snappily from troubles and stay zeroed in coming.

Individual Satisfaction changed over individuals continually witnessing a further raised position of individual satisfaction and fulfillment.

The Joint effort Among Movement and Lightening Advance and easing are naturally associated, each one designing up the other Mitigation Fills Progress When you are changed over, you will undoubtedly take action, set forth items, and work toward advance.

Progress Supports Mitigation Seeing improvement, at any rate of how little, can help easing and make up the conviction that you are looking great.

Set forth protests for Movement Portray clear, possible articles that give lightening and bearing to your development cycle.

Notice Achievements See and commendation your achievements in transit, which can likewise motivate you to keep on pushing ahead.

Methodology to Follow Movement and Remain Energized Ideal Setting Set Wise(Unequivocal, Quantifiable, possible, material, and Time-bound) protests that give clarity and mitigation to your movement interaction.

Separate It Hole greater articles into additional unobtrusive, more sensible advances.

arranging these accomplishments can uphold mitigation and give a sensation of progress.

Imagine Accomplishment: Make a cerebral picture of your substance.

Portrayal can redesign easing and work on your gift. Search for incitement Enclose yourself with moving distinctions, stories, or explanations that resonate with your items and values.

Stay Capable: Deal your articles with a reputation who can think of you as mindful and extend help and comfort.

Notice Progress Don't hang on until you show up at the last ideal to celebrate.

Fete and compensate yourself for each step of advance. Overcoming Obstacles to Movement and Motivation Misgiving about Frustration Fathom that accidents are significant for the trip.

Embrace frustration as learning an entryway. Non Appearance of Bearing If you are feeling lost, return to your articles and survey your prerequisites.

Searching for straightforwardness can reignite lightning. Breakdown Stay adjusted by adjusting your preliminaries and appreciating conventional respites.

Dealing with oneself is a veterinarian for staying aware of easing. outer Tensions Accepting external tensions are affecting your mitigation, put down places to pause and pass your musts on to individuals around you.

Negative tone-Talk Challenge negative contemplations and discipline them with positive statements that help mitigation.

The Tenacious Progression station To completely embrace the cooperative energy of advance and lightning, foster a terrible headway standpoint Flexibility Encourage the ability to snappily get back from incidents, understanding that they're wandering landmarks to progress.

Consistency Foster irremovable affirmation to keep on pushing forward, for sure despite troubles.

Improvement Course Embrace an improvement knowledge that welcomes new problems and entryways for education and upgrade.

Rigidity Be versatile and open to change, understanding that it continually prompts advancement and progress.

Energy Adapt your items to your endlessly advantages. Energy can be areas of strength for lightning.

End Embrace the Trip of Tenacious Headway Pursuing an exceptional life, following movement and remaining ceaselessly awakened are the underpinnings of accomplishment.

By fostering the cooperation among headway and lightning, you can make a diurnal reality stacked up with a patient turn of events, fulfillment, and the bleak confirmation to arrange your dreams.

Thus, set out on this trip of limitless development, worked up by troubling mitigation, and let it lead you to an unborn spilling over with accomplishments and unlimited possible issues.

2. Spreading out Sensible Goals:

Fanning Out Reasonable Focuses on: The Way to Doable Dreams

Goals are the compass that coordinates our journey all through regular day to day existence, with the exception of setting reasonable targets is the best approach to ensuring those dreams become a reality. Reasonable objectives look like areas of strength for the whereupon we develop the support of our desires. They outfit us with a sensible aide and an internal compass. Could we explore the specialty of defining reasonable objectives and how it plans for doable dreams.

- The Power of Reasonable Targets

Laying out reasonable objectives incorporates portraying clear, plausible spotlights that are agreed with your abilities, resources, and time goals. Here is the explanation it's so fundamental:

Motivation: Reasonable targets are impelling considering the way that they are reachable. They keep you not permanently set up to make progress.

Clearness: They give clarity by representing authoritatively the way that you truly need to achieve your goals, making it more direct to remain on track.

Sureness: Achieving reasonable objectives upholds your assurance and confidence in your abilities, pushing you toward more prominent dreams.

Resource The leaders: They help you with managing your resources beneficially in light of the fact that you're not seeking after inaccessible goals.

- The Art of Setting Reasonable Targets

Describe Express Goals: Be clear about what you want to achieve. Indistinct objectives make it hard to measure progress.

Separate It: Hole greater targets into additional humble, more reasonable advances or accomplishments. This makes the journey less overwhelming.

Zero in on: Recognize which targets make a big difference to you and spotlight your energy on those first.

Time-Bound: Put down a point in the time range for achieving your objectives. This makes a need to hurry up an obligation.

Sensible Examination: Survey your continuous abilities, resources, and requirements things being what they are. Make an effort not to misconstrue what you can achieve in a given time span.

151

Flexibility: Be accessible to changing your objectives as conditions change. Versatility is major for adaptability.

- Benefits of Setting Reasonable Targets

Upheld Motivation: Achieving more unobtrusive, reasonable targets keeps your motivation high all through your journey.

Diminished Tension: Understanding that your objectives are achievable reduces strain and anxiety.

More noticeable Pride: More unassuming triumphs on the way add to a pride, driving you closer to your conclusive dreams.

Further created Focus: Setting reasonable targets helps you with staying aware of revolving around the central thing.

Overhauled Self-Reasonability: Progress in achieving reasonable objectives helps your confidence in your capacities, working on self-ampleness.

- Beating Troubles On the way

Disasters: Fathom that mishaps are a piece of any trip. As opposed to believing them to be disillusionments, view them as any entryways to learn and change your objectives.

Time Necessities: In case time objectives become an issue, return to your objectives and widen the course of occasions if significant. Remember, the outing is fundamentally all around as critical as the goal.

Resource Obstructions: Evaluate your resources reliably and find compelling fixes to work inside your cutoff points.

Burnout: Remain adjusted by finding a consistent speed and getting a charge out of respites when required. It's important to stay aware of your physical and mental success.

- The Amiability Among Want and Credibility

While setting reasonable targets is principal for progress, it's moreover huge not to permit them to confine your goal. Reasonable targets go about as wandering stones toward greater dreams, but they shouldn't restrict your vision.

Discovering some sort of concordance among want and realness is imperative to achieving importance.

- End: Investigating the Way to Feasible Dreams

In the phenomenal weaving of life, putting forth reasonable objectives looks like cross sectioning the strings of your dreams into a significant reality.

These objectives give plan and bearing, ensuring that you make predictable progress toward your desires. Review that dreams may be boundless, yet reasonable targets are the implies that lead you there.

Along these lines, embrace the specialty of laying out reasonable objectives as you set out on your trip of advancement and accomplishment.

Permit them to be the coordinating stars that light your direction and the motivation that incites you forward.

With reasonable objectives as your mates, you'll see that your dreams are desires as well as reachable genuine variables fit to be perceived.

3. Ways to remain Reliable:

Ways Of staying Solid: The Foundation of Trust and Achievement

Dependability is a quality that sets the establishment for trust, regard, and outcome in both individual and expert life. At the point when you're known as somebody who can be depended on, entryways open, connections fortify, and open doors flourish. To help you become and stay solid, here are a few vital standards and systems to consider.

1. Consistency is Critical

Consistency is the sign of unwavering quality. It implies conveying results and meeting responsibilities reliably, not simply once in a while. To stay predictable:

Put forth attainable objectives and cutoff times.
Keep away from overcommitting; just commitment what you can reasonably convey.
Lay out schedules and stick to them.

2. Successful Correspondence

Clear and open correspondence is significant for unwavering quality. To be solid in your correspondence:

Speak the truth about your capacities and limits.
Impart plainly and proactively. Try not to leave space for uncertainty.
Keep partners educated regarding any progressions or postponements expeditiously.

3. Focus on Using time productively

Powerful using time productively is fundamental for dependability. This is the way to work on around here:

Use schedules and daily agendas to remain coordinated.
Allot adequate time for undertakings and activities.
Keep away from tarrying; tackle assignments immediately.

4. Construct Trust Through Responsibility

Responsibility is a foundation of unwavering quality. To cultivate trust:

Acknowledge liability regarding your activities and responsibilities.
Recognize slip-ups and attempt to amend them.
Try not to rationalize; all things considered, center around arrangements.

5. Learn and Adjust

Staying dependable likewise includes persistent learning and transformation:
Remain current with industry patterns and best practices.
Be available to input and utilize it to get to the next level.
Embrace change and adjust to new conditions.

6. Oversee Assumptions

Obviously overseeing assumptions is imperative for unwavering quality. To actually do this:
Ensure others have a practical comprehension of what you can and can't convey.
Don't over promise to kindly; set reasonable assumptions.
Remain conservative but then exceed everyone's expectations whenever the situation allows.

7. Put down Stopping points

Keeping up with dependability requires defining limits:

Figure out how to say no when important to keep away from overcommitment.
Safeguard your own time and prosperity to guarantee you can reliably follow through on your responsibilities.

8. Embrace Versatility

Versatility is a fundamental part of unwavering quality. It implies returning from misfortunes and remaining focused on your objectives:

Foster a development outlook that perspectives challenges as any open doors for development.
Use misfortunes as growth opportunities and fuel for future achievement.

9. Nonstop Personal growth

Unwavering quality is a persistent excursion of personal development:
Put resources into individual and expert improvement to upgrade your abilities and capacities.

Remain inquisitive and open to new information and encounters.

10. Cultivate Dependability

Dependability and unwavering quality remain inseparable. To cultivate trust:
Be faithful to your responsibilities and values.
Keep up with secrecy and regard others' protection.
Fabricate solid connections in view of shared trust and regard.

11. Reflect and Assess

Customary self-reflection and assessment are fundamental for staying dependable:

Evaluate your presentation and unwavering quality routinely.
Distinguish regions for development and find proactive ways to address them.

12. Put forth Clear Objectives

Laying out clear and explicit objectives assists you with keeping on track and solid:
Characterize your targets and separate them into significant stages.
Measure progress and change your course on a case by case basis.

- End: The Dependability Benefit

Being known as a dependable individual is an important resource in all parts of life. It constructs trust, upgrades your standing, and opens ways to new open doors.

Whether you're taking a stab at outcome in your profession or trying to reinforce your own connections, dependability is the foundation whereupon you can construct a satisfying and prosperous life.

In this way, focus on these standards and methodologies, and watch as your unwavering quality turns into a main impetus for your prosperity and prosperity.

Chapter 8:

1. Beating Typical Challenges:

In the excursion of life, it's normal to experience deterrents, mishaps, and difficulties that test our versatility and assurance.

Part 8 is tied in with excelling at beating these normal troubles that life tosses our direction. A manual for vanquishing the common obstacles can at times feel unfavorable.

1. The Industriousness Challenge

Industriousness is the way to beating any hindrance. It's tied in with pushing through whenever difficulties arise and remaining focused on your objectives. When confronted with the industriousness challenge:

Reevaluate Misfortunes: Rather than considering difficulties to be disappointments, view them as any open doors to learn and move along.

Remain on track: Watch out for the award, and don't let interruptions or impermanent disappointments crash your advancement.

Look for Help: Rest on companions, family, guides, or an encouraging group of people when you really want support and inspiration.

2. The Time Usage Problem

Adjusting time is a consistent battle, however successful using time productively is an expertise worth dominating. To vanquish the time usage predicament:

Focus on Undertakings: Recognize the main errands and tackle them first.

Set Practical Cutoff times: Keep away from overcommitting and set attainable cutoff times for your assignments.

Figure out how to Say No: Occasionally, saying no is important to safeguard your time and needs.

3. The Certainty Emergency

An absence of certainty can be a huge barrier to advance. While confronting a certainty emergency:

Challenge Negative Self-Talk: Supplant self-uncertainty with positive certifications and faith in your capacities.

Observe Little Wins: Recognize and celebrate even minor accomplishments to support your certainty.

Persistent Learning: Put resources into personal growth and instruction to build your abilities and confidence.

4. The Choice Problem

Simply deciding, particularly significant ones, can dismay. To handle the choice issue:

Assemble Data: Settle on informed choices by gathering all important data and choices.

Look for Guidance: Talk with confided in tutors, companions, or specialists while confronting difficult decisions.

Pay attention to Your Gut feelings: In some cases, your premonition is your best aid. Trust yourself.

5. The Feeling of dread toward Disappointment

The feeling of dread toward disappointment can keep you away from facing challenges and chasing after your fantasies. To defeat it:

Shift Your Viewpoint: See disappointment as a venturing stone to progress, not as the stopping point.

Begin Little: Start with sensible difficulties and progressively move gradually up to greater objectives.

Remain Versatile: Develop flexibility to return quickly from disappointments more grounded and savvier.

6. The Dawdling Trap

- Dawdling can be an impressive foe. To get away from the dawdling trap:

Put forth Clear Objectives: Characterize your targets and break them into more modest, reasonable undertakings.

Lay out an Everyday practice: Make a day to day or week after week schedule that consolidates undertakings connected with your objectives.

Use Responsibility: Offer your objectives with somebody who can consider you responsible for your advancement.

7. The Pressure Issue

Stress is a typical trouble that influences both mental and actual prosperity. To deal with the pressure problem:

Practice Unwinding Procedures: Consolidate unwinding techniques like profound breathing, contemplation, or yoga into your everyday daily schedule.

Work-out Consistently: Active work is an incredible pressure minimizer, delivering endorphins that further develop mind-set.

Focus on Taking care of oneself: Commit time to taking care of oneself exercises that help you unwind and re-energize.

8. The Inspiration Challenge

- Remaining propelled long term can be a challenge. To vanquish the inspiration challenge:

Put forth Clear Objectives: Characterize your goals and why they make a difference to you. This lucidity can fuel your inspiration.

Track down Your Why: Find your more profound reason and enthusiasm that drives you to succeed.

- Imagine Achievement: Make a psychological picture of your prosperity to keep inspiration high.

9. The Burnout Fight

Burnout is an unavoidable trouble, particularly in the present high speed world. To win the burnout fight:

- Lay out Limits: Put down clear stopping points to safeguard your own time and prosperity.

Focus on Taking care of oneself: Focus on taking care of oneself and consistently participate in exercises that re-energize you.

- Figure out how to Delegate: Feel free to assignments and obligations when essential.

10. The Compulsiveness Catch 22

Compulsiveness can impede progress by setting ridiculous guidelines. To get away from the compulsiveness conundrum:

Embrace Flaw: Acknowledge that flawlessness is impossible, and take a stab at greatness all things considered.

Set Practical Guidelines: Characterize attainable objectives and be caring to yourself when you miss the mark.

- Observe Progress: Perceive and praise your accomplishments, regardless of how little.
- End: Dominating Life's Normal Troubles

In the amazing story of your life, Section 8 is tied in with overcoming the ordinary difficulties that test your guts.

It's an update that troubles are essential for the excursion, and with the right procedures, outlook, and assurance, you can defeat them.

171

Embrace these standards, and you'll observe that the impediments in your way are not road obstructions but rather venturing stones to a more brilliant and more refined future.

2. Managing A throbbing painfulness:

Overseeing A throbbing painfulness: Recovering Solace and Imperativeness

A pulsating torment, whether it's a dull throb or a sharp twinge, can be an unwanted friend in our regular routines. It has the ability to upset our schedules, influence our mind-set, and ruin our efficiency. Be that as it may, with the right methodologies and outlook, overseeing a throbbing painfulness isn't just imaginable yet can likewise prompt expanded solace and essentialness.

1. Grasp the Cause of Torment

The most important phase in actually overseeing torment is to grasp its source. Is it because of a new physical issue, constant condition, or unfortunate stance? Distinguishing the main driver decides the suitable way to deal with tormenting the executives.

2. Counsel a Medical care Proficient

In the event that the aggravation endures or declines, counseling a medical services professional is fundamental. They can analyze the issue, preclude any hidden ailments, and suggest reasonable medicines or treatments.

3. Torment Drug and Help

Over-the-counter pain killers can give transitory help from gentle to direct agony. Nonetheless, it's significant to utilize them as coordinated and not depend on them as a drawn out arrangement. For constant torment, counsel a medical care supplier for recommended medicine choices.

4. Non-intrusive treatment and Exercise

Active recuperation can be profoundly viable in overseeing and reducing torment. A certified actual specialist can make a customized practice program to reinforce muscles, further develop adaptability, and lessen torment. Normal, low-influence practices like swimming, yoga, or kendo can likewise assist with keeping up with portability and oversee uneasiness.

5. Intensity and Cold Treatment

Applying intensity or cold to the impacted region can give help from agony and irritation. Utilize a boiling water bottle, warming cushion, or steaming shower for sore muscles and joints, and apply ice packs to lessen enlarging and numb torment.

6. Stance and Ergonomics

Unfortunate stance, particularly whenever supported over significant stretches, can add to a throbbing painfulness. Focus on your stance, both while sitting and standing, and put resources into ergonomic furnishings and assistants to help your body's normal arrangement.

7. Stress Decrease and Unwinding Strategies

Stress can worsen torment and distress. Consolidate pressure decreases procedures like profound breathing, contemplation, and care into your everyday daily practice to assist with overseeing torment all the more really.

8. Rest and Rest

Sufficient rest is critical for the body's recuperating and recuperation processes. Guarantee you have an agreeable bedding and focus on quality rest to help with torment the executives.

9. Dietary Decisions

Integrate mitigating food sources into your eating routine, like organic products, vegetables, entire grains, and greasy fish wealthy in omega-3 unsaturated fats. These can assist with diminishing aggravation and mitigate torment.

10. Elective Treatments

Investigate elective treatments like needle therapy, knead treatment, chiropractic care, or home grown cures. These methodologies can give alleviation to certain people and supplement customary clinical medicines.

11. Mind-Body Association

Consider mind-body rehearsals like directed symbolism and biofeedback. These procedures can assist you with overseeing your body's reactions to torment and diminish its force.

12. Strong Organization

Construct an encouraging group of people of loved ones who can offer profound help during seasons of torment. Imparting your encounters and sentiments to others can assist you with adapting to torment all the more really.

13. Remain Dynamic and Locked in

While it's fundamental for rest when required, it is similarly critical to stay away from complete idleness. Take part in exercises you appreciate, regardless of whether you want to adjust them to oblige your aggravation. Remaining dynamic can work on your state of mind and in general prosperity.

14. Track Your Aggravation

Keep an aggravation journal to follow the seriousness, term, and triggers of your aggravation. This can assist you and your medical care supplier with better comprehending your condition and designer therapy in a like manner.

15. Acknowledgment and Variation

Acknowledge that living with some degree of agony might be a reality, however it doesn't need to characterize your life. Adjust to your conditions, track down ways of working around your restrictions, and spotlight on what you can do instead of what you can't.

End: Recovering Solace and Imperativeness

Overseeing a throbbing painfulness is an excursion that requires tolerance, constancy, and a comprehensive methodology.

By joining clinical guidance, way of life changes, and a positive outlook, you can recover solace and essentialness in your life.

Recollect that aggravation the executives isn't tied in with killing uneasiness altogether yet working on your personal satisfaction and keeping up with your general prosperity.

3. Carving out Opportunity and Space for Your 5-Minute Exercises:

Cutting Out A potential open door and Space for Your 5-Minute Activities

In the present high speed world, carving out the opportunity for exercise can be an overwhelming undertaking.

Notwithstanding, the magnificence of 5-minute activities lies in their accommodation and adaptability.

You don't require hours at the rec center to remain dynamic and sound; everything necessary is a little imagination and assurance to cut out a valuable open door and space for your short, powerful exercises.

1. Embrace the Force of Short Explodes

The possibility that you want to save a huge piece of time for practice is a typical misguided judgment.

Short explosions of actual work can be comparably compelling, while perhaps not all the more thus, in accomplishing wellbeing and wellness objectives.

Research has demonstrated the way that concise, extraordinary exercises can give huge advantages, including working on cardiovascular wellbeing, expanded digestion, and upgraded muscle tone.

2. Carve out Pockets of Opportunity

Search for pockets of time over the course of your day when you can crush in a 5-minute activity meeting. Here are a few models:

Morning Schedule: Begin your day with a fast arrangement of bodyweight practices like squats, push-ups, or boards.

Work Breaks: Rather than going after an espresso during your work break, complete a little exercise to recharge.

Television Ad Breaks: Utilize business breaks while staring at the television to sneak in almost no time of activity. You'll be astonished at how these short spans add up.

Prior to Bed: Integrate a short extending routine into your sleep time routine to loosen up your muscles and further develop rest quality.

3. Be Effective with Gear

You needn't bother with a completely prepared exercise center to get a decent exercise. Negligible hardware or even your body weight can do the trick. Consider putting resources into opposition groups, free weights, or a soundness ball for mixing it up and power in your 5-minute activities.

4. Utilize Applications and Online Assets

There's a wealth of wellness applications and online assets that offer speedy, directed exercises. These apparatuses can assist you with capitalizing on your 5-minute activity meetings by giving construction and assortment. Whether you incline toward yoga, HIIT, or strength preparing, there's an application or video for you.

5. Include Your Environmental factors

Integrate your current circumstance into your exercises. Utilize a solid seat for step-ups or plunges, a wall for wall-sits, or a ledge for slant push-ups. Your environmental elements can become significant activity props.

6. Consolidate Exercise with Everyday Errands

Incorporate activity with day to day assignments to save time and set out additional open doors for actual work. For instance:

Use the Stairwell: Pick steps rather than lifts or elevators whenever the situation allows.

Strolling Gatherings: On the off chance that you have a gathering with a partner, recommend a mobile gathering as opposed to sitting in a meeting room.

Dynamic Driving: If attainable, walk or bicycle to attempt to integrate practice into your day to day drive.

7. Focus on Assortment

The same old thing all the time wears out a person's soul likewise a vital part of effective 5-minute activities. Pivoting through various activities forestalls weariness and targets different muscle gatherings, guaranteeing a balanced exercise routine daily schedule.

8. Put forth Practical Objectives

Putting forth reachable wellness objectives can be a strong inspiration. Whether it's raising the quantity of push-ups you can do or working on your adaptability, having substantial goals for your 5-minute activities keeps you not set in stone.

9. Include Your Loved ones

Connect with your loved ones in your wellness process. Besides the fact that you persuade each other, however you can likewise make 5-minute activities a tomfoolery and social action.

10. Remain Reliable

Consistency is key with regards to receiving the rewards of 5-minute activities. Make it an everyday propensity, and you'll before long notification enhancements in your solidarity, perseverance, and by and large wellness.

11. Pay attention to Your Body

While consistency is significant, it's similarly critical to pay attention to your body and stay away from overexertion or injury. On the off chance that you're feeling exhausted or encountering inconvenience, it's OK to enjoy some time off or change your activities.

12. Observe Your Accomplishments

Try not to misjudge the force of praising your triumphs, regardless of how little they might appear. Every 5-minute activity meeting is a stage toward better wellbeing, and recognizing your endeavors can support inspiration and build up your obligation to remaining dynamic.

- Decision: A Better You in Only 5 Minutes

In the fantastic plan of life, 5 minutes might appear to be a small detail within a bigger landscape, yet those concise snapshots of activity can fundamentally affect your general prosperity.

By cutting out open doors and space for your 5-minute activities, you're not just adopting a proactive strategy to your well being yet in addition sending a strong message that wellness is feasible and versatile to your bustling way of life.

In this way, hold onto those 5-minute windows, capitalize on them, and watch as they amount to a better, more fiery you.

Chapter 9:

Instances of Defeating Difficulty:

Life is an excursion loaded up with its reasonable portion of difficulties and misfortunes. In this chapter, we dive into the motivating accounts of people who have dealt with misfortune directly, showing exceptional flexibility, assurance, and mental fortitude.

These genuine models act as encouraging signs, outlining that affliction can be vanquished and change can emerge from the haziest of times.

1. Helen Keller - Win over Tangible Disconnection

Helen Keller, conceived hard of hearing and visually impaired in the late nineteenth hundred years, confronted unrivaled affliction.

With the resolute backing of her instructor, Anne Sullivan, Keller conquered her separation and figured out how to impart through gesture based communication and Braille. Her unyielding soul and tireless quest for information drove her to turn into a creator, teacher, and political dissident, motivating incalculable others with inabilities to try the impossible.

2. Malala Yousafzai - Hero of Schooling

Malala Yousafzai, a Pakistani young lady, opposed the Taliban's severe rule in her old neighborhood to advocate for young ladies' schooling.

She endured a shot to the head and, instead of being quieted, used her nerve racking experience to turn into a worldwide supporter for training and young ladies' freedoms. Malala's mental fortitude procured her the Nobel Harmony Prize, making her the most youthful ever laureate.

3. Nelson Mandela - From Detainee to President

Nelson Mandela, an enemy of politically-sanctioned racial segregation progressive, burned through 27 years in jail for his activism against racial isolation in South Africa. Upon his delivery, he pardoned his oppressors and worked vigorously to calmly destroy politically-sanctioned racial segregation.

Mandela's versatility and obligation to compromise made him an image of expectation and an impetus for change, in the long run prompting his political race as South Africa's most memorable dark president.

4. Stephen Selling - The Force of the Brain

Physicist Stephen Peddling confronted the impressive test of amyotrophic horizontal sclerosis (ALS), a crippling neurological sickness. Regardless of losing his capacity to move and speak, Selling proceeded with his pivotal examination in hypothetical physical science and turned into a smash hit creator. His life exemplified the boundless capability of the human psyche and soul, even despite significant actual misfortune.

5. Oprah Winfrey - Ascending from Affliction

Oprah Winfrey's initial life was set apart by neediness, misuse, and affliction. She conquered these difficulties to become perhaps one of the most powerful medium tycoons on the planet. Through her syndicated program, generosity, and backing for social issues, Oprah has enlivened millions to transcend their conditions and seek after their fantasies.

6. Viktor Frankl - Viewing as Importance in Anguish

Holocaust survivor Viktor Frankl persevered through the revolutions of Auschwitz and other inhumane imprisonments. His encounters drove him to create logotherapy, a psychotherapeutic methodology fixated on seeing significance in misery.

Frankl's significant bits of knowledge into the human soul advise us that even in the most obscure of times, we have the ability to track down reason and trust.

7. J.K. Rowling - From Dismissal to Scholarly Peculiarity

Prior to accomplishing worldwide popularity as the creator of the Harry Potter series, J.K. Rowling confronted various dismissals from distributors.

She drove forward through destitution and individual battles, utilizing her encounters to make a universe of sorcery and marvel. Rowling's excursion from misfortune to progress is a demonstration of the groundbreaking influence of narrating and strength.

8. Bethany Hamilton - Riding Past Impediments

Bethany Hamilton, an expert surfer, lost her arm in a shark assault at 13 years old. Unflinching, she got back to serious riding simply a month after the occurrence.

Her assurance and uplifting perspective made her a motivation to competitors around the world, demonstrating that actual limits need not characterize one's true capacity.

9. Thomas Edison - The Illumination of Development

Thomas Edison experienced endless disappointments and difficulties while fostering the glowing light. He broadly commented, "I have not fizzled. I've quite recently found 10,000 different ways that won't work." Edison's tireless quest for development and refusal to surrender eventually prompted perhaps the most groundbreaking creation ever.

10. Anne Plain - A Voice In the midst of Haziness

Anne Plain, a Jewish young lady in stowing away during The Second Great War, chronicled her encounters in her journal. In spite of the unbelievable difficulties she confronted, her compositions have contacted the hearts of millions and revealed insight into the human limit with respect to versatility and trust even notwithstanding affliction.

End: Win Over Affliction

accounts of people who conquered affliction advise us that the human soul is strikingly versatile. These models act as encouraging signs, outlining that misfortune, however testing, can be an impetus for development, empathy, and positive change.

They rouse us to stand up to our own difficulties with boldness and assurance, realizing that even in our most obscure minutes, there is the potential for change and win.

2. Rousing Stories of 40+ Wellness Change:

Energizing Accounts of 40+ Wellbeing Change

The excursion to health isn't restricted by age; as a matter of fact, it frequently takes on an entirely different aspect for those in their 40s and then some.

These motivating accounts of people who left on extraordinary wellbeing ventures sometime down the road demonstrate that focusing on your wellbeing and prosperity is rarely past the point of no return.

1. Angela's Staggering Weight reduction
Excursion

Angela, a 45-year-old mother of two, concluded
it was the ideal opportunity for a change. She
had battled with her weight for quite a long time,
yet the tipping point came when her PCP
communicated worries about her wellbeing.

Angela began little, consolidating day to day
5-minute exercises and step by step going with
better food decisions. After some time, her
consistency paid off. She shed abundant weight,
acquired certainty, and even ran her most
memorable long distance race at 50 years old.
Angela's story advises us that sincerely and
steadily, huge health changes are conceivable.

2. John's Noteworthy Wellness Change

At 48, John ended up driving an inactive way of
life, troubled by business related pressure and
medical problems. Worried about his future, he
chose to assume responsibility for his well

being. John began by strolling 5 minutes every day, step by step expanding his movement level. He consolidated strength preparing, adaptability works out, and better dietary patterns into his daily practice.

Strikingly, by his 50th birthday celebration, John had changed his body, shed pounds, and essentially diminished his gamble factors for constant sicknesses. His story fills in as evidence that focusing on wellness and rolling out significant improvements is rarely past the point of no return.

3. Lisa's Excursion to Mental and Close to home Prosperity

In her late 40s, Lisa encountered a progression of individual difficulties that left her inclination overpowered and sincerely depleted. She understood that her psychological and close to home prosperity were essentially as significant as her actual wellbeing.

Lisa looked for treatment and embraced care and reflection rehearses. Through steady taking care of oneself, she continuously discovered a sense of harmony and flexibility. Today, at 52, Lisa emanates energy and fills in to act as an illustration of how focusing on mental and close to home health can prompt extraordinary self-improvement.

4. Imprint's Experiences in Comprehensive Wellbeing

At 42, Imprint chose to adopt an all encompassing strategy to his prosperity. He integrated a reasonable eating regimen, standard activity, contemplation, and a pledge to getting sufficient rest into his everyday daily schedule.

Imprint's groundbreaking process prompted a better body, expanded energy levels, and a seriously satisfying life. His story highlights the meaning of exhaustive health rehearses in accomplishing essentialness and equilibrium, even in middle age.

5. Sarah's Astounding Profession Change

Sarah, in her mid 50s, had gone through a long time in high-stress work that had negatively affected her wellbeing.

Perceiving the requirement for a change, she chose to seek after her energy for comprehensive nourishment and health. Sarah returned to school and procured affirmations in sustenance and health training.

Today, she helps other people carry on with better existences and has found a satisfying second profession. Her story is a demonstration of the chance of rehashing and tracking down reason in one's 40s and then some.

End: Embracing Wellbeing Change at Whatever stage in life

These awakening accounts of people in their 40s and past exhibit that wellbeing change isn't restricted by age.

Whether it's accomplishing actual wellness, working on mental and close to home prosperity, embracing all encompassing wellbeing, or making a profession change, the consistent idea is the force of assurance, constancy, and the conviction that positive change is feasible.

These accounts encourage us to focus on our wellbeing and prosperity, regardless of where we are in life's excursion, and to perceive that the way to health is available to all who decide to live on it.

3. Decision: A Better, More joyful You:

Choice: A Superior More Cheerful
Life is a perplexing trap of decisions, every choice forming our way and impacting our prosperity. With regards to direction, it's not just about exploring life's intersection; it's tied in with creating a superior, more cheerful variant of ourselves. In this investigation of the significant effect of choices, we divulge the extraordinary force of decision.

1. The Choice to Focus on Taking care of oneself

The choice to focus on taking care of oneself is a statement of self-esteem. It includes defining limits, saying no when fundamental, and devoting time to feed your physical, mental, and profound prosperity.

At the point when taking care of oneself turns into a cognizant decision, it makes ready for further developed wellbeing, diminished pressure, and a more noteworthy feeling of delight and satisfaction.

2. The Choice to Embrace Inspiration

Deciding to embrace inspiration is a choice to see the world through a more splendid focal point. It includes rethinking negative considerations, rehearsing appreciation, and looking for open doors for development in each experience.

The gradually expanding influence of this choice is a daily existence loaded up with trust, strength, and a getting through feeling of bliss.

3. The Choice to Seek after Enthusiasm

Choosing to seek after your enthusiasm is a certification of your interesting reason and wants. It implies thinking for even a second to lean on your instinct, in any event, when it leads you down an eccentric way.

At the point when energy directs your decisions, you track down satisfaction, a feeling of direction, and the delight that comes from making every moment count.

4. The Choice to Develop Strength

Versatility is a choice to quickly return more grounded from life's difficulties. It includes recognizing difficulties as any open doors for development, adjusting to change, and keeping an uplifting perspective even in misfortune.

The choice to develop flexibility engages you to confront challenges with mental fortitude and rise up out of them with recently discovered strength and bliss.

5. The Choice to Sustain Connections

The choice to support connections perceives the significant effect of human associations on our prosperity. It includes putting time and exertion in building significant bonds with family, companions, and friends and family. At the point when connections are fundamentally important, they become a wellspring of help, love, and colossal bliss.

6. The Choice to Embrace Nonstop Learning

Deciding to embrace nonstop learning is a pledge to individual and scholarly development. It implies looking for new information, securing new abilities, and staying open to change and advancement.

This choice prompts a day to day existence wealthy in encounters, self-awareness, and the delight of finding new skylines.

7. The Choice to Lay out Intense Objectives

Laying out striking objectives is a choice to push your limits and try the impossible. It includes characterizing your desires, separating them into significant stages, and chasing after them with enduring assurance.

At the point when you go with the decision to put forth and seek after aggressive objectives, you open your maximum capacity and experience the elating delight of accomplishment.

8. The Choice to Practice Appreciation

Rehearsing appreciation is a choice to track down satisfaction right now. It includes recognizing the favors in your day to day existence, regardless of how little, and communicating appreciation for them.

The choice to rehearse appreciation changes your point of view, permitting you to track down euphoria and satisfaction in the present time and place.

9. The Choice to Excuse and Give up

Deciding to pardon and give up is a choice to deliver the weights of hatred and outrage. It includes perceiving that clutching past complaints just obstructs your own bliss.

At the point when you go with this decision, you free yourself from the heaviness of antagonism and discover a sense of reconciliation and bliss in pardoning.

10. The Choice to really Live

The choice to live really is a statement of self-acknowledgement. It implies embracing your actual self, blemishes and all, and adjusting your decisions to your guiding principle and convictions.

At the point when you pick credibility, you carry on with a day to day existence that is certified, satisfying, and consistent with who you are, giving you a significant feeling of pleasure and inward harmony.

End: The Force of Your Decisions

Every choice you make is a brushstroke on the material of your life, molding the work of art that is your remarkable excursion.

At the point when you deliberately pick taking care of oneself, inspiration, enthusiasm, flexibility, supporting connections, ceaseless learning, strong objectives, appreciation, pardoning, and legitimacy, you portray a superior, more upbeat you.

The force of your decisions lies in their nearby effect as well as in their capacity to shape the substance of your reality into one loaded up with reason, bliss, and significant happiness. Your life is a material trusting that your strokes of decision will make a show-stopper of satisfaction and satisfaction.

conclusion:

Embracing a Long period of 5-Minute Wellness:

Choice: A Superior, More Happy You

Life is a multifaceted trap of decisions, every choice forming our way and affecting our prosperity. With regards to independent direction, it's not only about exploring life's junction; it's tied in with creating a superior, more euphoric form of ourselves.

In this investigation of the significant effect of choices, we divulge the groundbreaking force of decision.

1. The Choice to Focus on Taking care of oneself

The choice to focus on taking care of oneself is a statement of self-esteem. It includes defining limits, saying no when vital, and committing time to sustain your physical, mental, and profound prosperity.

At the point when taking care of oneself turns into a cognizant decision, it prepares for further developed wellbeing, diminished pressure, and a more prominent feeling of delight and satisfaction.

2. The Choice to Embrace Inspiration

Deciding to embrace inspiration is a choice to see the world through a more brilliant focal point. It includes reexamining negative contemplations, rehearsing appreciation, and looking for open doors for development in each experience.

The expanding influence of this choice is a daily existence loaded up with trust, versatility, and a persevering through feeling of bliss.

3. The Choice to Seek after Energy

Choosing to seek after your energy is a certification of your remarkable reason and wants. It implies actually thinking about depending on your instinct, in any event, when it leads you down an offbeat way. At the point when energy directs your decisions, you track down satisfaction, a feeling of direction, and the delight that comes from living life to the fullest.

4. The Choice to Develop Versatility

Versatility is a choice to return more grounded from life's difficulties. It includes recognizing mishaps as any open doors for development, adjusting to change, and keeping an uplifting perspective even in difficulty.

The choice to develop flexibility engages you to confront hardships with fortitude and rise out of them with recently discovered strength and bliss.

5. The Choice to Sustain Connections

The choice to sustain connections perceives the significant effect of human associations on our prosperity. It includes putting time and exertion in building significant bonds with family, companions, and friends and family.

At the point when connections are vital, they become a wellspring of help, love, and enormous euphoria.

6. The Choice to Embrace Constant Learning

Deciding to embrace ceaseless learning is a pledge to individual and scholarly development. It implies looking for new information, getting new abilities, and staying open to change and development.

This choice prompts a day to day existence wealthy in encounters, self-improvement, and the delight of finding new skylines.

7. The Choice to Put forth Strong Objectives

Defining strong objectives is a choice to push your limits and try the impossible. It includes characterizing your goals, separating them into significant stages, and chasing after them with faithful assurance.

At the point when you go with the decision to put forth and seek after aggressive objectives, you open your maximum capacity and experience the elating delight of accomplishment.

8. The Choice to Practice Appreciation

Rehearsing appreciation is a choice to track down bliss right now. It includes recognizing the endowments in your day to day existence, regardless of how little, and communicating appreciation for them. The choice to rehearse appreciation changes your viewpoint, permitting you to track down euphoria and satisfaction in the present time and place.

9. The Choice to Pardon and Give up

Deciding to pardon and give up is a choice to deliver the weights of disdain and outrage. It includes perceiving that clutching past complaints just upsets your own bliss. At the point when you pursue this decision, you free yourself from the heaviness of pessimism and discover a sense of reconciliation and bliss in pardoning.

10. The Choice to genuinely Live

The choice to live genuinely is a statement of self-acknowledgement. It implies embracing your actual self, blemishes and all, and adjusting your decisions to your guiding principle and convictions.

At the point when you pick credibility, you carry on with a daily existence that is certifiable, satisfying, and consistent with who you are, giving you a significant feeling of pleasure and inward harmony.

- End: The Force of Your Decisions

Every choice you make is a brushstroke on the material of your life, molding the work of art that is your extraordinary excursion.

At the point when you deliberately pick taking care of oneself, inspiration, energy, flexibility, sustaining connections, nonstop learning, striking objectives, appreciation, pardoning, and credibility, you portray a superior, more blissful you.

The force of your decisions lies in their nearby effect as well as in their capacity to shape the quintessence of your reality into one loaded up with reason, satisfaction, and significant happiness.

Your life is a material trusting that your strokes of decision will make a work of art of happiness and satisfaction.